Independent ANCC Med Surg Exam Study Guide 2027–2028:

650 Practice Questions with Detailed Rationales for the Medical-Surgical Nursing Certification

AF879954

Caldwell Abiodun

📚 STUDY GUIDE BONUS MATERIAL

🎧 Full Audio Edition
Access the complete book in audio format
Ideal for learning during travel, workouts, or downtime
Stay productive even when you're not in the mood to read

📱 Digital Flashcards
Fast and effective revision tool
Strengthen memory of important concepts
Study anytime, wherever you are

⚡ Quick & Easy Access
No sign-up needed
Compatible with all devices
Smooth and instant usability

📍 *Access all bonus content on Page 12*

Author Introduction

Medical-surgical nursing forms the backbone of acute care practice, requiring clinical precision, adaptability, and comprehensive knowledge across diverse patient populations. The Medical-Surgical Nursing Certification (CMSRN®) credential recognizes registered nurses who demonstrate advanced competence in caring for adult patients with complex medical and surgical conditions. This study guide has been developed by an experienced medical-surgical nurse leader in collaboration with a team of clinical educators, acute care specialists, and certification preparation experts committed to supporting candidates in achieving CMSRN® success.

The lead author brings extensive experience in hospital-based adult care, interdisciplinary coordination, patient education, and quality improvement initiatives. Medical-surgical nurses manage a broad spectrum of conditions—from cardiovascular and respiratory disorders to endocrine, neurological, gastrointestinal, and postoperative complications. Success in this specialty demands strong assessment skills, effective prioritization, evidence-based intervention, and safe medication administration. This guide reflects those professional expectations by translating real-world acute care expertise into structured, exam-focused preparation aligned with the standards established by the Medical-Surgical Nursing Certification Board (MSNCB).

Working collaboratively, the contributing team conducted a comprehensive review of the CMSRN® examination content outline to ensure thorough coverage of its major domains. These include physiologic health conditions, professional practice concepts, patient safety, and interdisciplinary collaboration. Each chapter integrates pathophysiology, pharmacology, nursing interventions, and patient education strategies, reinforcing both conceptual understanding and applied clinical reasoning essential for exam performance.

Recognizing that CMSRN® candidates are often actively practicing nurses balancing demanding patient assignments, this study guide is intentionally structured for clarity and efficiency. Complex disease processes and treatment modalities are presented in organized, accessible language without sacrificing clinical depth. Scenario-based practice questions, prioritization frameworks, and focused review tools are incorporated to strengthen retention and build exam-day confidence.

Above all, this resource reflects deep respect for the essential role medical-surgical nurses play in delivering safe, high-quality care to adult patients. Earning the CMSRN® credential represents more than passing an examination—it signifies clinical expertise, professional dedication, and a commitment to excellence in acute care nursing. It is the sincere intention of the author and collaborative team that this guide serves as both a comprehensive pathway to certification success and a reaffirmation of the meaningful impact medical-surgical nurses have within today's healthcare systems.

Table of Content

Disclaimer

MEDSURG-BC® is a registered trademark of the American Nurses Credentialing Center. This publication is an independent study tool and is not affiliated with or endorsed by ANCC .

Chapter 1 – Assessment and Diagnosis

Assessment and diagnosis form the core of clinical judgment. Within the medical-surgical setting, nurses collect, analyze, and interpret a vast range of physiologic and psychosocial data to identify patient needs and actual or potential health problems. This process begins with systematic observation and continues through the integration of subjective and objective findings.

In practice, a thorough assessment involves establishing a **baseline of normal function**, recognizing variations that signal risk or disease, and applying critical reasoning to link findings to underlying pathophysiology. Nurses interpret data in the context of the individual's life stage, cultural background, comorbidities, and environment. Each piece of information—vital signs, laboratory values, physical examination, and reported symptoms—contributes to a pattern that supports the nursing diagnosis and subsequent plan of care.

A comprehensive database typically includes four components: **health history**, **physical examination**, **diagnostic testing results**, and **patient or caregiver input**. The health history focuses on the reason for seeking care, past medical and surgical experiences, medication use, allergies, and lifestyle habits. The physical examination proceeds from general inspection to focused system assessments, using inspection, palpation, percussion, and auscultation techniques. According to the provided material, accurate assessment relies on systematic sequencing—beginning with airway, breathing, and circulation before moving to region-specific evaluations.

Clinical Reasoning in Data Interpretation

Clinical reasoning transforms raw data into meaningful clinical information. Nurses apply pattern recognition to identify trends such as deteriorating oxygen saturation, progressive edema, or neurological changes. The ability to differentiate **normal compensatory responses** from **pathologic findings** is essential for early intervention.

For example, consider a postoperative patient whose heart rate increases and blood pressure declines. Through assessment and reasoning, the nurse interprets these findings not as simple anxiety but as possible hypovolemia. By correlating history, intake and output, and wound drainage, the nurse develops a prioritized diagnosis of "Deficient Fluid Volume" and notifies the interprofessional team promptly.

Diagnostic reasoning is guided by the **nursing process**: assess, diagnose, plan, implement, and evaluate. The diagnostic phase bridges assessment and intervention. It requires identifying both the problem and its related factors, distinguishing between *actual* and *risk* nursing diagnoses, and validating findings with the patient whenever possible.

The content emphasizes using standardized nursing terminology to ensure clear communication. Validated frameworks such as NANDA-I diagnostic categories allow nurses to articulate clinical judgments concisely and consistently. Accuracy in this step affects every subsequent domain of the exam, especially planning and evaluation.

Assessment Priorities Across Body Systems

In medical-surgical nursing, system-based assessments demand proficiency in detecting deviations that may signal instability.

- **Cardiovascular:** Evaluate perfusion through heart sounds, capillary refill, jugular venous distention, and peripheral pulses. Monitor for early signs of decreased cardiac output such as hypotension, cool extremities, or altered mental status.

- **Respiratory:** Observe effort, symmetry of chest expansion, breath sounds, and oxygenation indices. Identify risk for atelectasis or ventilator-associated complications.
- **Neurologic:** Perform level-of-consciousness checks, pupillary reactions, and motor strength assessments. Note changes that could indicate hypoxia, hypoglycemia, or stroke.
- **Gastrointestinal and Renal:** Assess intake, output, bowel patterns, and laboratory indicators of hydration and kidney function. Recognize nausea, distention, or reduced urine output as potential markers of imbalance or obstruction.
- **Integumentary and Musculoskeletal:** Inspect for pressure injuries, surgical wounds, edema, and mobility limitations that influence recovery.

Across all systems, assessment findings must be **documented objectively** and **communicated promptly** using SBAR or equivalent frameworks. The exam tests recognition of critical values and the nurse's prioritization response—distinguishing between findings requiring routine follow-up and those demanding immediate action.

Advanced Diagnostic Reasoning

Once assessment data are collected, the nurse engages in **analytic synthesis**—linking cues to patterns that support specific nursing diagnoses. Effective diagnostic reasoning integrates physiologic knowledge, patient preferences, and safety principles. The process begins with cue clustering—organizing signs and symptoms that appear related. From there, hypotheses are generated and tested against evidence.

For example, a patient admitted with dyspnea, fatigue, and peripheral edema may present with abnormal lung sounds and elevated jugular venous pressure. The nurse identifies a pattern consistent with impaired cardiac output, supported by diagnostic data such as low ejection fraction and weight gain. Validation of findings with objective tests ensures accuracy before interventions begin.

The *Medical-Surgical Nursing* reference emphasizes **dynamic reassessment**. Patient status is not static; subtle shifts in mental clarity, urinary output, or skin temperature can precede critical changes. Certification-level practice requires nurses to perform continuous evaluation rather than episodic checks, documenting updates and communicating emergent patterns rapidly.

Cultural and Psychosocial Considerations in Assessment

Comprehensive assessment extends beyond physiologic data. The patient's psychosocial, spiritual, and cultural dimensions directly affect health outcomes and compliance with treatment. Cultural awareness involves recognizing beliefs that shape health perceptions and decision-making. For example, attitudes toward pain expression, nutrition, or end-of-life care can vary across populations.

According to the reference material, culturally sensitive assessment begins by **establishing rapport** and asking open-ended questions. Nurses should avoid assumptions and instead invite patients to describe their perspectives on illness and care preferences. Inclusion of family or community members in assessment may be appropriate when consistent with patient wishes.

Psychosocial evaluation includes determining coping mechanisms, support systems, and emotional responses to illness. Anxiety, depression, and fear can alter physiological responses such as sleep patterns, immune function, and pain perception. By addressing these factors early, nurses enhance patient engagement and safety.

Prioritization and Critical Thinking

Prioritization is essential for safe and effective nursing care. The exam tests the ability to determine which assessment findings require **immediate action** versus those appropriate for later follow-up. Frameworks such as **ABCs (Airway, Breathing, Circulation)** and **Maslow's hierarchy of needs** guide prioritization decisions.

For instance, an oxygen saturation drop to 86% takes precedence over mild postoperative discomfort because airway compromise poses the greatest risk to survival. Similarly, a sudden change in mental status warrants rapid assessment for hypoxia, hypoglycemia, or stroke. Candidates are expected to interpret subtle clues and act within the nurse's scope before escalation.

Critical thinking supports prioritization through reflective questioning:

- What data are most significant to the patient's immediate safety?
- Which findings confirm or refute my current clinical impression?
- Have I validated abnormal results before implementing interventions?

The *Medical-Surgical Nursing* text reinforces the use of structured thinking strategies, such as concept mapping and clinical reasoning cycles, to organize and evaluate information. These skills are central to the exam's scenario-based questions that test practical judgment.

Case Example: Complex Assessment

A 68-year-old patient with chronic obstructive pulmonary disease (COPD) is admitted for worsening shortness of breath. Assessment reveals:

- Respiratory rate: 28 breaths/min, using accessory muscles
- Pulse oximetry: 88% on room air
- Heart rate: 118 beats/min
- Skin: cool, pale, and diaphoretic
- Breath sounds: diminished bilaterally with expiratory wheezes

The nurse correlates these findings with baseline data and identifies **ineffective breathing pattern** related to airflow obstruction and anxiety. Before implementing interventions, the nurse reassesses oxygen saturation with supplemental oxygen, positions the patient upright, and notifies the provider. Ongoing assessment includes monitoring for fatigue, increased work of breathing, and changes in arterial blood gases.

This example illustrates the integration of physiologic data, clinical judgment, and prioritization. Certification-level nurses must demonstrate the ability to link symptoms with causes, anticipate complications, and collaborate effectively to restore stability.

Diagnostic Validation and Collaboration

Once potential nursing diagnoses are formed, **validation** ensures that interpretations are accurate and relevant. Validation involves verifying subjective and objective data with the patient, reviewing supporting evidence from diagnostic tests, and consulting with the interprofessional team when uncertainties arise. The nurse's role includes ensuring that identified problems are evidence-based rather than assumption-driven.

For instance, if a patient reports dizziness and weakness, validation requires checking orthostatic blood pressures, reviewing medication profiles, and examining laboratory results for electrolyte imbalances. Collaboration with physicians, pharmacists, and therapists refines the diagnosis and directs safe care planning.

According to the provided reference material, **shared validation** reduces errors and enhances patient safety. When findings appear inconsistent, nurses reexamine assessment data rather than fitting evidence to preconceived expectations. This iterative process distinguishes competent assessment from mere observation.

Documentation of validated data must be precise, objective, and timely. Charting by exception—recording only deviations from the norm—is acceptable only when baseline data are established and clearly defined. Otherwise, comprehensive recording of assessments supports communication and legal protection.

Use of Diagnostic Tests and Laboratory Interpretation

In the medical-surgical environment, diagnostic tests complement physical assessment. Nurses are expected to interpret laboratory and imaging data within clinical context. Abnormal values should never be considered in isolation. For example, elevated creatinine levels gain significance only when correlated with urine output, hydration status, and medication use.

Common categories of diagnostic data include:

- **Hematologic:** Complete blood count, coagulation profiles, and indicators of infection or anemia.
- **Metabolic:** Electrolytes, glucose, renal and liver function panels, reflecting systemic regulation.
- **Cardiopulmonary:** Arterial blood gases, cardiac enzymes, and imaging results that clarify oxygenation and perfusion.

Interpretation also extends to recognizing **critical values** requiring immediate notification. Nurses should know institutional policies regarding critical alert thresholds and appropriate escalation procedures.

Certification exam questions often present data clusters—vital signs, lab values, and symptoms—requiring synthesis into a single diagnosis. The ability to connect abnormal laboratory results to clinical manifestations is central to this domain.

Documentation Standards and Communication

Accurate documentation transforms individual assessments into a cohesive patient record. Effective communication depends on clarity, precision, and neutrality of language. The *Medical-Surgical Nursing* reference underscores that every chart entry should be factual, complete, and chronological. Avoiding vague descriptors such as "appears comfortable" strengthens reliability; instead, document observable findings like "reports pain 2/10, resting quietly with regular respirations."

Structured communication tools, such as **SBAR (Situation, Background, Assessment, Recommendation)**, improve consistency across care transitions. The nurse provides concise yet comprehensive summaries when handing off patients or escalating care. Documentation of interdisciplinary updates—such as physician rounds or consult notes—ensures continuity and shared accountability.

Legal and ethical standards demand that charting accurately reflects the care provided. Altering or omitting data compromises integrity and violates professional codes. When errors occur, single-line corrections with signature and date maintain transparency.

In the exam context, questions may test recognition of best documentation practices, confidentiality standards, and ethical handling of sensitive data.

End-of-Domain Summary and Exam Tips

Assessment and diagnosis together form the foundation upon which all other nursing functions rest. The nurse's capacity to identify problems early, interpret subtle changes, and validate findings determines patient outcomes.

Key takeaways include:

- Conduct holistic assessments integrating physiologic, psychosocial, and cultural data.
- Use structured reasoning to cluster findings and validate nursing diagnoses.
- Prioritize according to immediate safety using ABCs and Maslow's framework.
- Document clearly, using standardized terminology and timely entries.
- Maintain continuous reassessment—conditions evolve, and effective care depends on detecting trends before deterioration occurs.

For exam preparation, practice interpreting short clinical vignettes with incomplete data. Ask, "What is most urgent? What is the likely cause? What is the nurse's next best action?" Focusing on reasoning steps rather than memorized answers builds the adaptability required for scenario-based questions.

Access Audio file and Flashcards

Scan QR Code Below

Chapter 2 – Planning, Implementation, and Evaluation

Effective nursing care depends on translating assessment findings into safe, goal-directed plans that are both evidence-based and individualized. This domain reflects the operational stage of the nursing process: determining priorities, establishing outcomes, initiating interventions, and measuring responses to care.

Planning integrates **critical reasoning with resource management**. Nurses weigh physiologic urgency, patient preferences, and available support systems. Interventions are sequenced based on clinical need and potential for improvement. Each plan must align with standards of practice and institutional protocols, ensuring consistency with national safety guidelines.

The *Medical-Surgical Nursing* reference emphasizes that successful planning begins with **clear, measurable outcomes**. Goals should be specific, attainable, relevant, and time-bound. For instance, "Patient will maintain oxygen saturation above 94% on 2 L/min oxygen by nasal cannula within 2 hours" is a measurable short-term objective. Such specificity allows nurses to track progress and adjust interventions efficiently.

Planning also includes anticipating complications. Preventive measures—such as repositioning to reduce pressure injury risk or maintaining aseptic technique for catheter care—demonstrate proactive nursing practice that the exam will evaluate.

Establishing Priorities of Care

Priority setting differentiates professional nursing practice from task-based routines. The nurse determines what actions must occur immediately and which can be delegated or scheduled. This process relies on applying principles of urgency, potential for harm, and patient stability.

The hierarchy of priorities typically follows:

1. **Life-threatening conditions** (airway obstruction, respiratory failure, circulatory collapse).
2. **Safety and risk reduction** (fall prevention, infection control, medication accuracy).
3. **Physiologic needs** (nutrition, elimination, mobility).
4. **Psychological and social needs** (coping, family support, education).

In exam scenarios, you may encounter multiple abnormal findings—one requiring emergent attention. For example, a patient with postoperative pain, mild fever, and new onset shortness of breath demands airway and circulation management before analgesic administration. The correct decision sequence demonstrates mastery of clinical prioritization.

Care Planning and Goal Formulation

Comprehensive care planning transforms the nursing diagnosis into actionable outcomes. The *Medical-Surgical Nursing* text describes two primary goal types:

- **Short-term goals**, which focus on immediate stabilization or symptom relief.
- **Long-term goals**, which address restoration of function, adaptation to chronic illness, and self-management education.

Effective goals meet several essential criteria:

- **Specificity:** Defines the exact outcome expected (e.g., "Wound edges remain approximated with minimal drainage").

- **Measurability:** Identifies how progress will be evaluated (e.g., "Pain score ≤3/10 within one hour after medication").
- **Realism:** Considers patient condition and available resources.
- **Time orientation:** Establishes a clear timeframe for expected results.

Each nursing diagnosis should have corresponding goals and interventions, ensuring continuity between assessment, planning, and implementation. Collaboration with the patient enhances adherence—plans that reflect personal preferences yield higher success rates.

In practice and on the exam, questions often test recognition of **the most appropriate goal** given the patient's stage of recovery. For example, immediately postoperatively, "maintain patent airway" supersedes "demonstrate deep breathing exercises."

Interdisciplinary Collaboration and Delegation

Implementation extends beyond individual nursing actions. It involves **coordination within the healthcare team** to deliver holistic, efficient care. Collaboration means engaging physicians, pharmacists, therapists, dietitians, and social workers to meet the complex needs of medical-surgical patients.

The reference material highlights **communication clarity** as the cornerstone of collaboration. Shared documentation systems, interdisciplinary rounds, and standardized care pathways promote unity of effort. The nurse often acts as liaison, translating patient goals into coordinated actions.

Delegation is another critical skill tested in this domain. Effective delegation adheres to the "Five Rights":

1. Right task
2. Right circumstance
3. Right person
4. Right direction or communication
5. Right supervision or evaluation

The registered nurse remains accountable for overall outcomes even when tasks are delegated. Understanding scope of practice distinctions between licensed and unlicensed personnel ensures both safety and compliance. On the exam, questions may ask which tasks can be delegated—for example, vital signs collection versus patient teaching—and which require RN assessment or evaluation.

Clinical Intervention Strategies

Implementation transforms the written plan into measurable action. Every nursing intervention must be purposeful, evidence-based, and responsive to ongoing assessment data. The *Medical-Surgical Nursing* reference underscores the principle of **clinical adaptability**—modifying interventions as the patient's condition evolves.

Examples of evidence-informed interventions include:

- Administering oxygen therapy while continuously monitoring saturation and respiratory effort.
- Maintaining intravenous access for fluid resuscitation, verifying site patency, and adjusting rate as ordered.

- Supporting mobility by encouraging gradual ambulation to prevent venous stasis and respiratory compromise.
- Using aseptic technique during wound care to minimize infection risk.

Each intervention carries both physiological and psychosocial dimensions. For instance, pain management includes not only pharmacologic administration but also relaxation, guided imagery, and environmental adjustments. The nurse's empathetic communication reinforces trust and compliance.

Implementation also includes **education**—a primary nursing responsibility. Teaching patients and families about procedures, medications, and discharge planning fosters independence and reduces readmissions. Certification candidates must demonstrate ability to adapt teaching methods to literacy level, cultural background, and readiness to learn.

Patient Safety and Risk Reduction

Safety forms the ethical and professional foundation of nursing care. This includes preventing harm through vigilant monitoring, adherence to protocols, and identification of hazards. Common safety principles reinforced in the exam include:

- **Infection control:** Hand hygiene, sterile field maintenance, and isolation precautions.
- **Medication safety:** Applying the "six rights" (right patient, drug, dose, route, time, documentation) and checking for allergies or interactions.
- **Fall prevention:** Implementing mobility aids, call light accessibility, and environmental checks.
- **Equipment verification:** Ensuring infusion pumps, monitors, and oxygen systems function correctly.

The *Medical-Surgical Nursing* material integrates national safety benchmarks such as sentinel event prevention, accurate patient identification, and surgical site verification.

Scenario-based questions often test the nurse's recognition of **early warning signs**—for example, detecting infiltration at an IV site before complications, or noting subtle neurological decline following head injury. Demonstrating proactive safety vigilance indicates advanced competence.

Evaluation of Outcomes

Evaluation closes the nursing process loop. It determines whether the goals established during planning have been met and whether interventions achieved desired results. Evaluation is not a final step but an **ongoing cycle of reflection and adjustment**.

Key components of effective evaluation include:

- **Data comparison:** Reviewing new assessment findings against established baselines.
- **Outcome measurement:** Determining if short-term and long-term goals were met, partially met, or unmet.
- **Reassessment:** Revising the care plan based on current patient status.
- **Collaboration:** Communicating results and modifications to the healthcare team.

When goals are not met, nurses analyze contributing factors—such as inadequate adherence, unforeseen complications, or inappropriate interventions. The revised plan then integrates improved strategies and education.

For instance, if a patient's postoperative pain remains uncontrolled despite medication, the nurse reassesses timing, dosage, and nonpharmacologic options, collaborating with the provider to adjust the regimen.

Certification-level questions may present incomplete data, requiring interpretation of whether interventions were effective or if the plan must change.

Case Example: Evaluating Complex Outcomes

A patient recovering from abdominal surgery exhibits stable vital signs but remains reluctant to ambulate. Despite multiple reminders, the patient reports pain and fatigue. The nurse reassesses pain management effectiveness, confirms analgesic timing, and applies motivational interviewing to identify emotional barriers. After adjusting the schedule to provide analgesia 30 minutes before ambulation and encouraging gradual pacing, the patient successfully completes short hallway walks without distress.

This scenario demonstrates adaptive evaluation: reassessing underlying factors, modifying interventions, and documenting improved functional outcomes. It reflects the exam's emphasis on **evaluation as continuous quality improvement** rather than static completion.

Outcome evaluation also encompasses patient satisfaction, comprehension of discharge instructions, and ability to self-manage chronic conditions. In medical-surgical nursing, success is measured not solely by physiologic stability but by patient confidence in sustaining health behaviors after discharge.

Integration of Evidence-Based Practice

Evidence-based practice (EBP) ensures that nursing care decisions rely on current, validated research integrated with clinical expertise and patient preferences. The *Medical-Surgical Nursing* reference underscores that the medical-surgical nurse must actively appraise literature, participate in quality improvement initiatives, and adapt interventions based on evolving standards of care.

Implementation of EBP follows a structured model:

1. **Ask** a focused clinical question.
2. **Search** for the best available evidence.
3. **Appraise** the strength and relevance of findings.
4. **Apply** evidence to clinical decision-making.
5. **Evaluate** outcomes and disseminate results.

For example, in preventing catheter-associated urinary tract infections, evidence supports removing indwelling catheters as soon as possible, ensuring aseptic insertion, and maintaining a closed drainage system. Translating this knowledge into daily practice reduces infection rates and improves patient outcomes.

On the exam, expect questions that assess your ability to identify which intervention best reflects evidence-based standards—such as choosing incentive spirometry over bed rest for postoperative pulmonary prevention.

EBP also connects to policy and education: nurses must advocate for guideline updates, participate in audits, and mentor peers in adopting research-supported methods.

Care Coordination and Continuity

Modern medical-surgical nursing extends beyond the inpatient setting. Effective care coordination ensures continuity across acute, rehabilitation, and community environments. The nurse functions as the **central communicator**, linking physicians, allied professionals, and caregivers to maintain a seamless care experience.

According to the reference material, coordination includes:

- **Transition planning:** Ensuring discharge readiness, medication reconciliation, and patient education.
- **Resource management:** Connecting patients with financial, social, and rehabilitative support.
- **Follow-up care:** Facilitating home health visits, telehealth follow-ups, and outpatient appointments.

Care coordination requires anticipating barriers—such as limited

Care Coordination and Continuity

Care coordination requires anticipating barriers—such as limited mobility, financial hardship, or lack of caregiver support—that may prevent adherence to the treatment plan. Nurses use communication skills to bridge these gaps, promoting safe transitions between settings

Continuity of care is sustained through structured documentation and communication methods. Tools such as discharge summaries, medication lists, and referral notes must be accurate, timely, and accessible. The nurse confirms patient comprehension by applying the *teach-back* technique, asking the patient to restate instructions in their own words.

In the exam, questions often involve care transitions: for example, identifying which action best supports safe discharge of a postoperative patient with new diabetes. The correct response usually integrates patient teaching, verification of understanding, and coordination with follow-up resources rather than simple task completion.

Care coordination also embodies **advocacy**. Nurses advocate for patients unable to voice their needs, ensuring equitable access to care regardless of cultural, social, or linguistic barriers. This holistic approach defines excellence in medical-surgical nursing.

Interprofessional Collaboration and Communication

The medical-surgical environment functions through teamwork. Effective collaboration requires mutual respect, clarity of roles, and shared decision-making. The *Medical-Surgical Nursing* reference highlights interprofessional collaboration as a dynamic exchange where each member contributes expertise toward patient-centered goals.

Nurses coordinate daily interactions among physicians, therapists, dietitians, and case managers, translating medical terminology into actionable information for patients and families. Structured rounding models—such as interdisciplinary bedside rounds—improve outcomes by aligning goals and minimizing duplication of effort.

Communication failures remain a leading cause of adverse events. Nurses must practice assertive but professional dialogue using frameworks like SBAR to report patient changes. For example, when a postoperative patient's heart rate increases suddenly, clear, concise communication enables rapid physician response. The exam tests this skill through scenario questions emphasizing prioritization, documentation, and escalation.

Effective collaboration also includes conflict management. Nurses balance advocacy for patient safety with respect for hierarchy, ensuring concerns are voiced constructively. This professional maturity demonstrates readiness for certification-level responsibility.

Quality Improvement and Performance Evaluation

Evaluation at the systems level involves analyzing care outcomes across patient populations to identify opportunities for improvement. Quality improvement (QI) initiatives often focus on reducing complications, enhancing satisfaction, or improving efficiency.

Examples include monitoring rates of hospital-acquired infections, medication errors, or readmissions. When trends are identified, the nurse contributes to root-cause analysis and develops action plans—such as revising procedures, increasing staff education, or updating clinical pathways.

The *Medical-Surgical Nursing* text notes that continuous QI aligns directly with patient safety initiatives like the Magnet Recognition Program and National Database of Nursing Quality Indicators. Understanding these frameworks reinforces professionalism and demonstrates that certification extends beyond individual competence to system-level impact.

In exam scenarios, you may be asked which response demonstrates engagement in QI—for example, participating in a falls prevention committee or reporting near misses to improve safety tracking. The correct choice always reflects proactive, evidence-informed participation rather than passive observation.

End-of-Domain Summary and Exam Tips

Domain II synthesizes the art and science of nursing implementation. Successful candidates demonstrate the ability to plan intelligently, act decisively, and evaluate continuously.

Key points to retain:

- **Plan with precision:** Define measurable, time-bound goals tailored to each patient.
- **Implement with intention:** Use evidence-based interventions that prioritize safety and collaboration.
- **Evaluate adaptively:** Modify care plans in response to outcomes and evolving conditions.
- **Document meticulously:** Record what was done, the patient's response, and next steps.
- **Collaborate consistently:** Communicate clearly across disciplines and advocate for continuity.

Chapter 3 – Professional Role

The professional role domain encompasses the ethical, legal, and leadership responsibilities that define nursing beyond clinical skills. The medical-surgical nurse functions as a decision-maker, patient advocate, and role model for safe, compassionate care. This domain reflects the nurse's accountability to patients, colleagues, and society through adherence to established codes of ethics and professional standards.

According to the reference material, the **core values** underpinning professional nursing include altruism, integrity, human dignity, and social justice. These values guide decision-making when clinical situations are complex or morally ambiguous.

Professional role mastery requires self-awareness and continuous professional growth. Nurses are expected to evaluate their practice, seek feedback, and participate in lifelong learning. Certification signifies not only competency but also commitment to evidence-informed leadership and ethical stewardship of patient trust.

Ethical Principles in Practice

Ethics guide every aspect of nursing care. Key principles emphasized in the exam include:

- **Autonomy:** Respecting the patient's right to make informed choices. Nurses must provide information without coercion and honor decisions even when they differ from personal beliefs.
- **Beneficence:** Acting in the patient's best interest through compassion and competence.
- **Nonmaleficence:** Avoiding harm by maintaining vigilance, accuracy, and empathy.
- **Justice:** Ensuring equitable care regardless of background, culture, or socioeconomic status.
- **Fidelity and Veracity:** Remaining faithful to commitments and communicating truthfully with patients and colleagues.

Ethical decision-making often requires balancing competing principles. For example, maintaining autonomy may conflict with beneficence when a patient refuses a lifesaving procedure. The *Medical-Surgical Nursing* text advises applying ethical frameworks such as the **ANA Code of Ethics** and consulting ethics committees for complex dilemmas.

The exam may present case-based questions testing recognition of ethical conflicts and appropriate actions—such as how to proceed when a family demands treatment contrary to the patient's advance directive. The correct response prioritizes the patient's expressed wishes while ensuring compassionate explanation to all parties.

Legal and Professional Accountability

Professional accountability ensures that nursing practice aligns with legal standards and institutional policies. Nurses are responsible for their actions, decisions, and documentation. The *Medical-Surgical Nursing* reference highlights several key aspects of legal responsibility:

1. **Scope of Practice:** Defined by state nurse practice acts and institutional job descriptions. Nurses must perform only those duties for which they are educated and licensed.
2. **Informed Consent:** The nurse verifies that the patient has received adequate information, understands the procedure, and voluntarily consents. While physicians obtain consent, nurses serve as advocates by confirming comprehension and reporting concerns.

3. **Confidentiality:** Protected under privacy regulations, requiring careful management of verbal and electronic communication.
4. **Delegation and Supervision:** The RN remains legally accountable for delegated tasks, ensuring that each activity is appropriate to the skill level of the delegatee.
5. **Documentation:** Accurate records serve as legal evidence of care provided.

Negligence, malpractice, and failure to follow standards of care can result in disciplinary or legal action. The exam often tests understanding of **liability** and **risk prevention**. For instance, identifying when to report a change in condition or when to complete an incident report demonstrates legal awareness.

Leadership and Professional Development

Leadership in medical-surgical nursing extends beyond managerial roles—it represents a mindset of accountability, mentorship, and continuous improvement. Effective leaders cultivate trust, communicate transparently, and foster collaboration across disciplines.

The reference material identifies leadership competencies such as **decision-making**, **conflict resolution**, and **team motivation**. Nurses demonstrate leadership when they precept new staff, coordinate care efficiently, or participate in policy development.

Professional development includes pursuing specialty certification, attending continuing education programs, and engaging in reflective practice. Nurses maintain competence through self-assessment and participation in peer review.

Leadership also encompasses **advocacy**—championing patient rights and promoting safe work environments. When resource shortages, ethical dilemmas, or unsafe practices arise, the nurse leads by voicing concerns through appropriate channels and proposing constructive solutions.

Patient and Family Education

Education is both a legal obligation and a professional hallmark of nursing. Medical-surgical nurses empower patients and families by providing the knowledge and skills necessary to manage illness and recovery effectively. According to the *Medical-Surgical Nursing* reference, successful teaching depends on clear communication, assessment of learning needs, and evaluation of understanding.

The teaching process includes:

1. **Assessment:** Determining readiness to learn, preferred learning styles, literacy level, and potential barriers.
2. **Planning:** Establishing achievable learning outcomes, such as demonstrating proper wound care or understanding medication schedules.
3. **Implementation:** Delivering education using visual aids, demonstrations, and teach-back methods.
4. **Evaluation:** Verifying comprehension by observing return demonstrations or having the learner restate key concepts.

Education is ongoing—it begins on admission and continues through discharge and follow-up care. Nurses must tailor instruction to the patient's cognitive, cultural, and emotional context. For example, providing written materials in the patient's preferred language and ensuring comprehension through interpretation services reflect cultural competence.

The exam frequently presents teaching scenarios requiring selection of the most effective or ethical approach, emphasizing clarity, timing, and verification.

Cultural Competence and Diversity

Cultural competence enables nurses to deliver care that respects and integrates individual beliefs, values, and traditions. The *Medical-Surgical Nursing* text stresses that culture influences health behaviors, perceptions of illness, and expectations of care.

Culturally competent care requires:

- **Self-awareness:** Recognizing one's own values and potential biases.
- **Knowledge:** Understanding cultural variations in communication, family structure, and health practices.
- **Skill:** Adapting care to accommodate cultural and linguistic needs without stereotyping.
- **Desire:** Demonstrating genuine respect and curiosity toward diverse backgrounds.

Examples include adjusting dietary teaching to honor religious restrictions, incorporating family in decision-making when culturally appropriate, and using certified interpreters rather than family members for translation.

In exam scenarios, the culturally sensitive answer usually demonstrates respect, nonjudgment, and individualized care—never assumptions or dismissive language.

Advocacy and Professional Influence

Advocacy defines the nurse's responsibility to protect patient rights and ensure that healthcare decisions align with the patient's values and preferences. This may involve clarifying information, addressing ethical conflicts, or intervening when safety is compromised.

The *Medical-Surgical Nursing* reference identifies three key dimensions of advocacy:

1. **Patient-Centered:** Promoting autonomy, privacy, and informed consent.
2. **Professional:** Upholding nursing standards and participating in policy development.
3. **Community and Systemic:** Supporting initiatives that improve access, quality, and equity of care.

Effective advocacy requires confidence and communication. Nurses must articulate concerns clearly, citing policy or evidence to support recommendations. For example, advocating for adequate pain management or early mobilization demonstrates leadership grounded in evidence and ethics.

In the exam, advocacy questions often focus on **assertive communication**—choosing statements that express concern respectfully while safeguarding patient welfare. The correct choice prioritizes the patient's needs, even if it challenges hierarchy.

Chapter 4 – Practice Questions

Questions (1-100)

Q1. A nurse assesses a patient with suspected heart failure. Which finding best supports fluid volume overload?

A. Dry mucous membranes
B. Jugular vein distension
C. Bradycardia
D. Hypotension

Q2. During lung auscultation, fine crackles are noted at the bases. What is the most likely cause?

A. Airway obstruction
B. Atelectasis or fluid in alveoli
C. Bronchospasm
D. Pleural friction rub

Q3. Which assessment finding requires immediate action in a patient with pneumonia?

A. Productive cough
B. Respiratory rate of 28/min
C. SpO_2 84% on room air
D. Fever of 101°F

Q4. A nurse palpates a bounding carotid pulse. Which condition is most consistent with this finding?

A. Hypovolemia
B. Aortic regurgitation
C. Heart block
D. Mitral stenosis

Q5. Which step should the nurse perform first when assessing a new patient?

A. Physical examination
B. Focused system review
C. Collect health history data
D. Obtain diagnostic test results

Q6. During neurological assessment, unequal pupils (3 mm right, 6 mm left) are noted. What should the nurse do first?

A. Document and recheck in 30 minutes
B. Notify the provider immediately
C. Check for dehydration
D. Continue with assessment

Q7. A nurse notes bilateral pitting edema in a patient's lower legs. What is the likely mechanism?

A. Decreased capillary permeability
B. Increased plasma oncotic pressure
C. Increased hydrostatic pressure
D. Lymphatic hyperactivity

Q8. When auscultating the heart, the nurse identifies an S3 gallop. What does this sound usually indicate?

A. Pulmonary embolism
B. Early diastolic filling due to heart failure
C. Mitral valve stenosis
D. Normal sound in adults

Q9. In performing abdominal assessment, the nurse auscultates before palpating. Why?

A. To detect rigidity first

B. To avoid altering bowel sounds
C. To assess for pain response
D. To check for rebound tenderness

Q10. Which assessment best indicates effective pain control?
A. Patient reports "better" pain
B. HR and BP return to baseline
C. Patient appears relaxed
D. Nurse observes no grimacing

Q11. When assessing hydration, which finding supports fluid volume deficit?
A. Crackles in lungs
B. Bounding pulses
C. Dry oral mucosa
D. Elevated jugular veins

Q12. Which laboratory value most directly correlates with renal function assessment?
A. AST
B. Creatinine
C. Bilirubin
D. Lipase

Q13. A diabetic patient reports numbness in the feet. Which assessment is most appropriate?
A. Babinski reflex
B. Monofilament test
C. Romberg test
D. Mini-Mental exam

Q14. What is the nurse's priority when performing a mental status exam?
A. Assess language fluency
B. Evaluate orientation to person, place, time
C. Test cranial nerve VII
D. Examine reflex responses

Q15. Which finding in a patient with COPD warrants immediate reporting?
A. Barrel chest
B. Clubbing of fingers
C. Respiratory rate 10/min
D. Use of accessory muscles

Q16. A nurse notes crackles that do not clear after coughing. What condition is suspected?
A. Atelectasis
B. Chronic bronchitis
C. Pulmonary edema
D. Upper airway obstruction

Q17. Which pulse site is preferred for assessing circulation to the lower extremities?
A. Carotid
B. Radial
C. Dorsalis pedis
D. Brachial

Q18. During assessment, a nurse detects a systolic murmur at the left sternal border. What tool helps confirm its nature?
A. Reflex hammer
B. Pulse oximeter
C. Echocardiogram

D. Spirometer

Q19. Which action is essential before performing a head-to-toe assessment?

A. Ask about allergies
B. Explain the procedure to the patient
C. Obtain physician consent
D. Prepare diagnostic equipment

Q20. When inspecting a wound, the nurse notes yellow drainage with foul odor. Which type of exudate is this?

A. Serous
B. Serosanguineous
C. Purulent
D. Sanguineous

Q21. Which assessment technique is used to evaluate liver size?

A. Palpation
B. Auscultation
C. Percussion
D. Inspection

Q22. A nurse finds a patient's skin turgor poor and mucous membranes dry. Which condition is most likely?

A. Fluid volume excess
B. Dehydration
C. Hyponatremia
D. Hypothermia

Q23. During cardiac assessment, a displaced apical impulse is palpated lateral to the midclavicular line. What does this indicate?

A. Right ventricular hypertrophy
B. Left ventricular enlargement
C. Pericardial effusion
D. Pulmonary embolism

Q24. A nurse percusses a dull sound over the left lower lung base. What does this most likely suggest?

A. Pleural effusion
B. Pneumothorax
C. Emphysema
D. Bronchospasm

Q25. Which assessment finding best indicates adequate tissue perfusion?

A. Pale nail beds
B. Capillary refill under 2 seconds
C. Cyanotic lips
D. Cool extremities

Q26. When assessing bowel sounds, the nurse hears none after one minute. What is the appropriate action?

A. Document as absent
B. Continue auscultation for five minutes
C. Begin palpation
D. Notify provider immediately

Q27. Which position optimizes lung expansion during respiratory assessment?

A. Supine
B. Semi-Fowler's

C. Trendelenburg
D. Lithotomy

Q28. Which finding in a diabetic patient suggests peripheral arterial disease?
A. Bounding pedal pulses
B. Hair loss on lower legs
C. Warm, moist skin
D. Rapid capillary refill

Q29. While examining the thyroid, a nurse notes enlargement that moves with swallowing. What is the best next action?
A. Notify provider immediately
B. Palpate gently for nodules or tenderness
C. Apply firm pressure
D. Begin carotid palpation

Q30. A patient with chronic anemia presents with spoon-shaped nails (koilonychia). Which underlying process explains this?
A. Iron deficiency
B. Vitamin B_{12} excess
C. Hypercalcemia
D. Dehydration

Q31. Which assessment finding supports hypocalcemia?
A. Positive Chvostek's sign
B. Bradycardia
C. Flaccid muscles
D. Hypoactive reflexes

Q32. During eye assessment, unequal pupil constriction after light exposure is observed. What does this suggest?
A. Normal variation
B. Cranial nerve III impairment
C. Dehydration
D. Cataract

Q33. Which assessment data are essential before administering a loop diuretic?
A. Blood glucose
B. Serum potassium and blood pressure
C. Urinalysis
D. Hemoglobin

Q34. A patient reports pain rated 8/10 but shows no distress. What should the nurse do?
A. Reassure the patient
B. Administer analgesic as prescribed
C. Defer treatment
D. Ask family to confirm

Q35. Which sound is expected over the stomach during percussion?
A. Dullness
B. Resonance
C. Tympany
D. Flatness

Q36. A nurse finds a pressure injury with full-thickness skin loss exposing subcutaneous tissue. Which stage is this?
A. Stage I

B. Stage II
C. Stage III
D. Stage IV

Q37. During respiratory assessment, prolonged expiratory phase is noted. Which disorder does this suggest?

A. Asthma
B. Pneumonia
C. Pleural effusion
D. Pulmonary fibrosis

Q38. Which finding indicates effective peripheral circulation after leg surgery?

A. Absent pedal pulse
B. Pale, cool toes
C. Warm pink feet with palpable pulses
D. Capillary refill > 5 seconds

Q39. A patient's blood pressure changes from 130/80 supine to 100/60 standing. What is this called?

A. Orthostatic hypotension
B. Essential hypertension
C. Secondary hypertension
D. Pulse deficit

Q40. Which factor is most critical when formulating nursing diagnoses?

A. Physician's orders
B. Objective and subjective assessment data
C. Patient preferences
D. Diagnostic imaging results

Q41. Which finding indicates early hypoxia in a postoperative patient?

A. Cyanosis of lips
B. Restlessness and anxiety
C. Slow heart rate
D. Cool clammy skin

Q42. A nurse palpates a patient's abdomen and feels a pulsating midline mass. What is the best action?

A. Continue palpating for size
B. Document as normal finding
C. Apply pressure to assess tenderness
D. Auscultate for a bruit and stop palpation

Q43. When performing a neurologic exam, the nurse uses the Glasgow Coma Scale (GCS). Which component is included?

A. Pupillary response
B. Eye opening, verbal, and motor response
C. Pain perception only
D. Reflex testing

Q44. Which finding most supports the nursing diagnosis "Impaired gas exchange"?

A. Productive cough
B. SpO_2 86% on 4 L oxygen
C. Warm, dry skin
D. Heart rate 78 bpm

Q45. A nurse notes a new onset of confusion in an elderly patient. What is the first nursing action?

A. Assess oxygen saturation and glucose level

B. Notify physician immediately
C. Start IV fluids
D. Document and observe

Q46. Which cardiac assessment finding requires urgent evaluation?
A. Regular rhythm, rate 90 bpm
B. S4 heart sound in elderly
C. New murmur with chest pain
D. Occasional premature beat

Q47. What is the priority nursing assessment before giving digoxin?
A. Radial pulse for 30 seconds
B. Apical pulse for one full minute
C. Blood pressure in both arms
D. Oxygen saturation level

Q48. Which sign best differentiates venous from arterial insufficiency?
A. Dependent rubor
B. Absent pedal pulses
C. Brown skin discoloration near ankles
D. Cold pale feet

Q49. A nurse observes that a patient's blood pressure drops significantly after sitting up. Which system is most involved?
A. Respiratory
B. Cardiovascular autonomic regulation
C. Endocrine
D. Renal filtration

Q50. Which abnormal lung sound suggests airway narrowing from secretions?
A. Crackles
B. Rhonchi
C. Pleural rub
D. Vesicular sounds

Q51. During assessment, a nurse notes jugular vein distension at 45°. This finding indicates:
A. Dehydration
B. Right-sided heart failure
C. Hypotension
D. Pulmonary embolism

Q52. Which test evaluates sensory discrimination between two close touch points?
A. Graphesthesia
B. Romberg test
C. Stereognosis
D. Two-point discrimination

Q53. A nurse palpates crepitus around a chest tube insertion site. What does this signify?
A. Normal healing
B. Subcutaneous emphysema
C. Pleural effusion
D. Infection

Q54. Which assessment best reflects adequate renal perfusion after surgery?
A. Urine output 30 mL/hr or greater
B. Pale, dry skin
C. Rising serum creatinine

D. Absent bowel sounds

Q55. Which sign indicates positive Trousseau's sign?

A. Hand spasms during blood pressure cuff inflation
B. Facial twitching after tapping facial nerve
C. Tremor with eyes closed
D. Flaccid hand drop

Q56. A patient's skin is pale and cool with delayed capillary refill. What physiologic issue does this suggest?

A. Peripheral vasodilation
B. Decreased tissue perfusion
C. Elevated cardiac output
D. Local infection

Q57. During eye inspection, a white arc around the cornea is observed in an older adult. What is the interpretation?

A. Corneal ulcer
B. Arcus senilis, normal aging change
C. Cataract formation
D. Lipid keratopathy

Q58. When assessing cranial nerve VII (facial), the nurse asks the patient to:

A. Shrug shoulders and turn head
B. Stick out tongue midline
C. Smile, frown, and puff cheeks
D. Close eyes and identify scent

Q59. Which finding suggests increased intracranial pressure?

A. Pupils equal and reactive
B. Widened pulse pressure and bradycardia
C. Rapid, shallow respirations
D. Bounding peripheral pulses

Q60. A nurse notes a patient's radial pulse is irregular. What should be the next assessment step?

A. Measure apical pulse for one full minute
B. Record rate as irregular and continue
C. Count for 15 seconds and multiply by four
D. Palpate pedal pulse

Q61. Which assessment is most important for a patient taking furosemide?

A. Skin turgor
B. Apical pulse
C. Serum potassium and daily weight
D. Pupillary reaction

Q62. When percussing over the lungs, hyperresonance is heard. What condition is most consistent?

A. Pneumonia
B. Pulmonary edema
C. Emphysema
D. Pleural effusion

Q63. Which assessment step follows inspection in a complete physical exam?

A. Palpation
B. Percussion
C. Auscultation
D. Depends on system examined

Q64. A patient with liver disease presents with yellow sclera. This finding results from:
A. Carotenemia
B. Hyperbilirubinemia
C. Anemia
D. Vitamin deficiency
Q65. Which condition causes a fruity odor on a patient's breath?
A. Uremia
B. Liver failure
C. Diabetic ketoacidosis
D. Gastroesophageal reflux
Q66. During cardiac auscultation, the nurse hears a pericardial friction rub. What condition does this suggest?
A. Endocarditis
B. Pericarditis
C. Myocardial infarction
D. Valve stenosis
Q67. Which finding is characteristic of right-sided heart failure?
A. Pulmonary crackles
B. Jugular vein distension
C. Dyspnea at rest
D. Orthopnea
Q68. A nurse assessing a patient notes clubbing of the fingers. What underlying issue is most likely?
A. Chronic hypoxemia
B. Dehydration
C. Anemia
D. Vitamin deficiency
Q69. What is the best indicator of effective fluid resuscitation in shock?
A. Warm skin
B. Increased urine output
C. Strong peripheral pulses
D. Decreased anxiety
Q70. A patient with COPD has a barrel chest. This indicates:
A. Chronic hyperinflation of the lungs
B. Muscle wasting
C. Fluid retention
D. Pleural effusion
Q71. When assessing lymph nodes, which characteristic is most concerning?
A. Soft and movable
B. Hard and fixed
C. Small and tender
D. Mobile and round
Q72. Which cranial nerve controls swallowing and gag reflex?
A. Cranial nerve IX and X
B. Cranial nerve VII
C. Cranial nerve XI
D. Cranial nerve XII
Q73. A nurse auscultates bowel sounds every 15 seconds in all quadrants. How should this finding be documented?

A. Normal active bowel sounds
B. Hyperactive bowel sounds
C. Hypoactive bowel sounds
D. Absent bowel sounds

Q74. Which abnormal breath sound indicates partial airway obstruction by secretions or tissue swelling?

A. Stridor
B. Wheeze
C. Crackles
D. Pleural rub

Q75. Which pulse site is most accurate for infants?

A. Radial
B. Apical
C. Temporal
D. Brachial

Q76. A nurse notes dry, flaky skin with thickened nails. These findings most likely indicate:

A. Arterial insufficiency
B. Venous stasis
C. Dehydration
D. Peripheral neuropathy

Q77. Which test helps differentiate between conductive and sensorineural hearing loss?

A. Snellen test
B. Weber and Rinne tests
C. Romberg test
D. Whisper test

Q78. During assessment, the nurse notes a patient's lips are cherry red. What condition should be suspected?

A. Carbon monoxide poisoning
B. Hypoxia
C. Cyanosis
D. Anemia

Q79. A patient reports dizziness upon standing. Which nursing intervention is most appropriate?

A. Encourage rapid position changes
B. Assess orthostatic vital signs
C. Increase caffeine intake
D. Restrict fluids

Q80. Which finding requires immediate intervention during respiratory assessment?

A. Occasional cough
B. Respiratory rate 22/min
C. Use of accessory muscles with cyanosis
D. Breath sounds diminished at bases

Q81. Which patient finding indicates effective cardiac output?

A. Weak pulses and cool extremities
B. Alertness, warm skin, and adequate urine output
C. Decreased blood pressure
D. Cyanotic nail beds

Q82. A nurse assessing lung sounds notes coarse crackles in both bases. What is the most probable cause?

A. Alveolar fluid accumulation
B. Bronchospasm
C. Pleural thickening
D. Airway obstruction by foreign body

Q83. A patient reports pain radiating to the left arm and jaw. Which system should the nurse assess immediately?
A. Neurologic
B. Cardiac
C. Musculoskeletal
D. Respiratory

Q84. Which assessment data best reflect adequate oxygenation?
A. SpO_2 96% and pink nail beds
B. RR 10/min and lethargy
C. Cyanotic lips with SpO_2 92%
D. Pale conjunctiva

Q85. The nurse finds a patient with asymmetrical chest expansion. Which condition is most likely?
A. Asthma
B. Pneumothorax
C. Bronchitis
D. Heart failure

Q86. Which finding is associated with dehydration?
A. Bounding pulse
B. Elevated hematocrit
C. Crackles in lungs
D. Jugular vein distension

Q87. A nurse palpates the posterior tibial pulses and finds them weak. What should be the next step?
A. Elevate the legs
B. Document as normal
C. Apply warm compresses
D. Compare both sides and assess capillary refill

Q88. Which assessment technique is most reliable for detecting ascites?
A. Light palpation
B. Fluid wave test
C. Inspection of skin color
D. Auscultation for bruits

Q89. A nurse observes a patient with facial drooping and slurred speech. What is the priority assessment?
A. Level of consciousness
B. Grip strength
C. Blood glucose
D. Airway and oxygenation

Q90. When assessing an elderly patient, which skin change is expected?
A. Thickened dermis
B. Increased elasticity
C. Decreased turgor and fragile capillaries
D. Excess sebaceous activity

Q91. Which finding supports a diagnosis of anemia?
A. Ruddy facial color

B. Pale conjunctiva and fatigue
C. Bounding peripheral pulses
D. Elevated blood pressure

Q92. A nurse notes inspiratory wheezes in both lung fields. What condition is most likely?
A. Pulmonary embolism
B. Asthma
C. Pneumonia
D. Pleural effusion

Q93. Which lab value would the nurse expect in a patient with dehydration?
A. Low hematocrit
B. Decreased sodium
C. Elevated blood urea nitrogen (BUN)
D. Reduced osmolality

Q94. Which finding is consistent with hypokalemia?
A. Muscle weakness and irregular pulse
B. Tetany and hyperreflexia
C. Bradycardia and tremors
D. Bounding pulses and hypertension

Q95. During ear examination, the tympanic membrane appears bulging and erythematous. What does this suggest?
A. Serous otitis media
B. Acute otitis media infection
C. Tympanic membrane perforation
D. Cerumen impaction

Q96. Which physical assessment finding suggests chronic venous insufficiency?
A. Shiny, hairless legs
B. Brown discoloration near ankles
C. Diminished pedal pulses
D. Cold extremities

Q97. Which parameter best reflects adequate ventilation?
A. SpO_2 100%
B. $PaCO_2$ 40 mm Hg
C. Respiratory rate 28/min
D. pH 7.55

Q98. A patient's tongue appears smooth and beefy red. Which deficiency is most likely?
A. Iron
B. Vitamin B_{12}
C. Vitamin D
D. Calcium

Q99. A nurse percusses a dull note over the left lower posterior lung. Which follow-up assessment is indicated?
A. Check for pleural effusion
B. Evaluate for hyperinflation
C. Assess for pneumothorax
D. Test for stridor

Q100. Which nursing assessment supports a diagnosis of hypoglycemia?
A. Warm, dry skin and polyuria
B. Sweating, tremors, and confusion

C. Slow pulse and hypertension
D. Weight gain and fatigue

Answer key and Explanation (1-100)

Q1. Answer: B

Explanation: Jugular vein distension indicates increased central venous pressure, a hallmark of right-sided heart failure. It differentiates volume overload from dehydration. Dry mucous membranes indicate deficit, while bradycardia and hypotension may appear in shock but not classic hypervolemia.

Q2. Answer: B

Explanation: Fine crackles indicate air passing through fluid-filled or collapsed alveoli, common in pulmonary edema or atelectasis. Bronchospasm produces wheezes, and pleural friction rubs result from pleural inflammation, not intra-alveolar fluid.

Q3. Answer: C

Explanation: An SpO_2 of 84% signifies hypoxemia and requires urgent oxygen therapy. Tachypnea and fever are expected infection responses, while productive cough indicates airway clearance but not critical oxygen impairment.

Q4. Answer: B

Explanation: A bounding carotid pulse results from increased stroke volume and rapid ejection in aortic regurgitation. Hypovolemia would reduce amplitude, and heart block or mitral stenosis typically produce weaker, irregular pulses.

Q5. Answer: C

Explanation: Health history collection precedes physical assessment, establishing baseline understanding of patient conditions. This sequence follows ANA and Bates' guidelines emphasizing subjective data before objective examination to ensure patient-centered assessment.

Q6. Answer: B

Explanation: Anisocoria, particularly new or significant, indicates possible increased intracranial pressure or cranial nerve III compression. Prompt provider notification is essential. Rechecking alone delays critical neuro intervention.

Q7. Answer: C

Explanation: Edema from increased hydrostatic pressure occurs with right-sided heart failure or venous congestion. Reduced oncotic pressure also causes edema but typically generalized, not localized. Lymphatic obstruction produces non-pitting swelling.

Q8. Answer: B

Explanation: S3 reflects rapid ventricular filling against a dilated ventricle, commonly from left-sided heart failure. It is pathological in adults but normal in children or pregnancy. S4 appears in stiff ventricles, not dilated ones.

Q9. Answer: B

Explanation: Palpation stimulates peristalsis and can distort bowel sound interpretation. Bates' recommends auscultation first to maintain accurate assessment of intestinal motility. Palpation follows to assess organ size or tenderness.

Q10. Answer: B

Explanation: Physiologic markers such as normalized vital signs objectively verify pain relief. Subjective statements may be vague, and visual cues can mislead due to patient masking behaviors. Combining both enhances reliability.

Q11. Answer: C

Explanation: Dry mucous membranes reflect extracellular fluid loss. Crackles and jugular distension indicate overload, while bounding pulses occur in hypervolemia, not dehydration.

Q12. Answer: B

Explanation: Serum creatinine reflects glomerular filtration efficiency and renal function. Elevated levels signal renal impairment. AST and bilirubin assess liver function, while lipase indicates pancreatic injury.

Q13. Answer: B

Explanation: The monofilament test evaluates peripheral neuropathy by assessing tactile pressure sensation. It detects sensory loss early. Babinski tests motor tract function; Romberg assesses balance, not peripheral sensation.

Q14. Answer: B

Explanation: Orientation is foundational for cognitive assessment, indicating cerebral function and acute changes. Language and cranial nerve exams provide additional detail but do not supersede establishing orientation baseline.

Q15. Answer: C

Explanation: A respiratory rate of 10/min suggests hypoventilation and CO_2 retention in a COPD patient. Other findings are chronic adaptations and expected; bradypnea signals acute respiratory depression risk.

Q16. Answer: C

Explanation: Non-clearing crackles represent alveolar fluid from pulmonary edema. Crackles resolving with coughing suggest mucus plugging, typical in bronchitis. Atelectasis presents with diminished, not bubbly, sounds.

Q17. Answer: C

Explanation: The dorsalis pedis pulse assesses arterial perfusion to distal legs and feet. Weak or absent pulses indicate peripheral arterial disease. Carotid and radial pulses reflect central circulation instead.

Q18. Answer: C

Explanation: Echocardiography visualizes valve structure and flow patterns, confirming murmur etiology such as stenosis or regurgitation. Pulse oximetry measures oxygen saturation but not cardiac sound origins.

Q19. Answer: B

Explanation: Explaining the process fosters cooperation, reduces anxiety, and upholds informed participation per ANA ethical standards. Allergy checks and equipment preparation follow after consent and explanation.

Q20. Answer: C

Explanation: Purulent exudate indicates infection, characterized by yellow or green thick fluid with odor. Serous is clear, sanguineous is blood-tinged, and serosanguineous combines plasma and blood components.

Q21. Answer: C

Explanation: Percussion estimates liver span by identifying dullness over hepatic tissue. Palpation alone can detect tenderness but not boundaries. Auscultation and inspection reveal vascular or surface findings, not organ size. Proper percussion differentiates hepatomegaly from other right-upper-quadrant masses using tone variation between tympany and dullness.

Q22. Answer: B

Explanation: Poor skin turgor and dry mucosa indicate extracellular fluid loss causing dehydration. These findings stem from reduced interstitial volume. Hyponatremia may coexist but presents neurologically, not with classic dryness. Hypothermia alters perfusion rather than turgor. Assess vital signs and intake-output to confirm volume deficit severity.

Q23. Answer: B

Explanation: Lateral displacement of the apical impulse signals left ventricular hypertrophy or dilation, often from hypertension or heart failure. Right ventricular hypertrophy moves the impulse left sternal, not lateral. Pericardial effusion muffles sounds, while pulmonary embolism produces tachycardia, not anatomical displacement.

Q24. Answer: A

Explanation: Dullness on percussion occurs when fluid or consolidation replaces air, typical of pleural effusion. Pneumothorax yields hyperresonance; emphysema creates overly resonant sounds from trapped air. Bronchospasm affects airflow but not percussion tone. Correlate with decreased breath sounds and possible shortness of breath.

Q25. Answer: B

Explanation: Rapid capillary refill demonstrates sufficient arterial blood flow and oxygenation to peripheral tissues. Delayed refill, pallor, or coolness signal compromised perfusion due to hypovolemia or vasoconstriction. Cyanosis reflects severe desaturation. Evaluating refill complements pulse palpation to confirm circulatory effectiveness.

Q26. Answer: B

Explanation: True absence requires five full minutes of auscultation in each quadrant before classification. Transient hypoactive sounds may follow surgery or narcotics. Premature documentation could misrepresent peristaltic activity. Continue listening systematically before notifying provider of possible ileus or obstruction.

Q27. Answer: B

Explanation: The semi-Fowler's position elevates the head 30–45°, promoting diaphragmatic excursion and chest expansion, enhancing auscultation accuracy. Supine limits ventilation, Trendelenburg impairs breathing, and lithotomy suits pelvic exams. Proper positioning also aids oxygenation assessment and patient comfort.

Q28. Answer: B

Explanation: Loss of hair, shiny skin, and diminished pulses reflect chronic ischemia from arterial insufficiency. Bounding pulses and warmth indicate adequate or excess flow, not occlusion. Early identification prevents ulceration or amputation through vascular evaluation and glycemic control.

Q29. Answer: B

Explanation: A thyroid that rises with swallowing warrants gentle bilateral palpation to assess consistency and nodularity. Excessive pressure risks tissue injury or carotid stimulation. Movement with swallowing indicates thyroid origin, distinguishing it from neck masses. Report abnormal texture or asymmetry afterward.

Q30. Answer: A

Explanation: Koilonychia reflects long-term iron-deficiency anemia altering keratin formation in the nail bed. It accompanies fatigue and pallor. Vitamin B_{12} excess and dehydration do not cause nail deformities; hypercalcemia affects neuromuscular tone. Iron restoration reverses structural changes gradually.

Q31. Answer: A

Explanation: A positive Chvostek's sign—facial twitch after tapping—indicates neuromuscular irritability from low calcium. Hypocalcemia causes tetany and hyperreflexia, whereas bradycardia and flaccidity occur with electrolyte excess. Verify via serum calcium and address causes like hypoparathyroidism or renal failure.

Q32. Answer: B

Explanation: The oculomotor nerve (cranial III) mediates pupillary constriction; unequal reaction signals neurological damage or pressure on the nerve. Dehydration and cataracts affect clarity or tearing, not pupil symmetry. Prompt neuro evaluation prevents complications from intracranial lesions.

Q33. Answer: B

Explanation: Loop diuretics like furosemide can cause hypokalemia and hypotension. Assess potassium levels and baseline blood pressure to avoid arrhythmias or circulatory collapse. Blood glucose and hemoglobin provide context but are secondary for immediate safety.

Q34. Answer: B

Explanation: Pain is subjective; absence of behavioral cues does not negate severity. Administering ordered analgesia honors patient self-report consistent with ANA ethical standards. Objective confirmation or deferral undermines trust and can delay relief.

Q35. Answer: C

Explanation: Tympany arises from gas-filled structures such as the stomach or intestines, signifying normal air presence. Dullness suggests fluid or organ tissue, resonance occurs over lungs, and flatness indicates bone. Absent tympany may signal obstruction or mass.

Q36. Answer: C

Explanation: Stage III ulcers extend through dermis into subcutaneous fat but not muscle or bone. Stage I shows redness, II partial-thickness, and IV deep exposure of muscle or bone. Accurate staging guides wound management and documentation for continuity of care.

Q37. Answer: A

Explanation: Asthma causes airway narrowing, prolonging expiration as trapped air escapes slowly. Pneumonia presents with crackles, pleural effusion with dullness, and fibrosis with decreased compliance, not extended expiration. Assess for wheezing and monitor peak flow.

Q38. Answer: C

Explanation: Warm, pink skin and palpable distal pulses confirm adequate arterial flow. Delayed refill, pallor, or coolness signal ischemia requiring urgent evaluation. Continuous assessment prevents postoperative vascular compromise such as compartment syndrome or thrombosis.

Q39. Answer: A

Explanation: A drop of ≥20 mm Hg systolic or ≥10 mm Hg diastolic upon standing defines orthostatic hypotension, indicating impaired autonomic or volume regulation. Hypertension involves elevation, and pulse deficit refers to radial-apical differences. Evaluate medications and hydration.

Q40. Answer: B

Explanation: Accurate nursing diagnoses derive from comprehensive assessment combining subjective symptoms and objective findings per ANA Standard 2. Physician orders inform treatment but not problem identification. Integrating patient input follows after establishing valid, data-supported nursing judgments.

Q41. Answer: B

Explanation: Restlessness and anxiety are early neurologic signs of hypoxia as the brain experiences oxygen deprivation first. Cyanosis is a late manifestation. Bradycardia and cool skin occur as hypoxia progresses to circulatory collapse. Prompt oxygen assessment prevents deterioration.

Q42. Answer: D

Explanation: A pulsating abdominal mass suggests possible aortic aneurysm. The nurse should stop palpation immediately to prevent rupture and auscultate gently for bruits. Pressure or deep palpation risks tearing. Documenting as normal would delay critical evaluation.

Q43. Answer: B

Explanation: The GCS measures level of consciousness using eye, verbal, and motor responses, scoring 3–15. It excludes pupillary size and reflexes. Lower scores indicate deeper coma. Frequent GCS monitoring aids early detection of neurologic deterioration.

Q44. Answer: B

Explanation: Low oxygen saturation despite supplemental oxygen reflects alveolar-capillary impairment. Productive cough and normal heart rate may coexist but do not confirm gas exchange deficits. Hypoxia assessment directs interventions like positioning or ventilation adjustments for correction.

Q45. Answer: A

Explanation: Sudden confusion often results from hypoxia or hypoglycemia. Assessment of oxygen and glucose provides rapid, reversible clues. Immediate notification follows if abnormal. Documentation without evaluation risks missing treatable acute changes, including delirium onset.

Q46. Answer: C

Explanation: A new murmur accompanying chest pain may signal valvular rupture or endocarditis, demanding immediate investigation. S4 can be age-related, and occasional premature beats are benign. Prompt cardiac workup ensures prevention of acute mechanical complications.

Q47. Answer: B
Explanation: Digoxin slows conduction through the AV node; checking apical pulse for a full minute prevents dosing in bradycardia (<60 bpm). Radial measurement is unreliable for rhythm irregularities. Blood pressure and oxygen aid context but not dose safety.
Q48. Answer: C
Explanation: Chronic venous insufficiency causes brown pigmentation from hemosiderin deposition. Arterial insufficiency produces pallor, coolness, and absent pulses. Dependent rubor reflects severe arterial disease. Recognizing skin changes aids accurate vascular assessment and targeted care.
Q49. Answer: B
Explanation: Postural or orthostatic hypotension results from impaired autonomic cardiovascular compensation to positional change, leading to venous pooling. Respiratory and renal systems influence oxygenation and volume but not immediate pressure shifts. Assess hydration and medication side effects.
Q50. Answer: B
Explanation: Rhonchi are low-pitched, snoring sounds caused by airflow through large airways obstructed by mucus. Crackles stem from alveolar fluid, pleural rubs from pleural inflammation, and vesicular sounds are normal. Suctioning or coughing may clear rhonchi effectively.
Q51. Answer: B
Explanation: Jugular vein distension when upright reflects elevated central venous pressure from right ventricular failure. Dehydration and hypotension reduce venous filling, while pulmonary embolism causes acute dyspnea but not sustained venous distension. Monitor for edema and hepatomegaly.
Q52. Answer: D
Explanation: Two-point discrimination measures parietal lobe sensory cortex function by assessing the minimal distance between distinct touches. Graphesthesia evaluates recognition of writing, and stereognosis identifies objects by touch. Romberg examines balance, not tactile discrimination.
Q53. Answer: B
Explanation: Crepitus, or crackling under the skin, results from air leakage into subcutaneous tissue—subcutaneous emphysema. It may indicate tube displacement or air leak. Infection causes redness and warmth but not crackling sensation. Notify provider for evaluation.
Q54. Answer: A
Explanation: Consistent urine output ≥30 mL/hr shows sufficient renal blood flow and function. Decreased output signals hypovolemia or renal ischemia. Creatinine elevation and pallor indicate delayed detection of renal compromise. Early monitoring ensures circulatory adequacy.
Q55. Answer: A
Explanation: Trousseau's sign appears when ischemia from BP cuff inflation triggers carpal spasms, revealing latent tetany from hypocalcemia. It results from increased neuromuscular excitability. Chvostek's sign involves facial twitching, while tremors and flaccidity reflect other neurologic or electrolyte disorders unrelated to calcium deficit.
Q56. Answer: B
Explanation: Pale, cool skin and delayed refill indicate reduced arterial perfusion due to hypovolemia or vasoconstriction. Vasodilation would cause warmth and flushing, while infection produces localized redness. Early identification of poor perfusion prevents ischemic tissue damage or shock progression.
Q57. Answer: B
Explanation: Arcus senilis is a benign white ring from lipid deposits in corneal margins common in aging. It does not impair vision or signal disease in older adults. Corneal ulcers and cataracts alter clarity, while keratopathy involves opacity and pain.
Q58. Answer: C

Explanation: Cranial nerve VII controls facial expressions; asking to smile, frown, and puff cheeks evaluates motor symmetry. Shoulder shrug tests CN XI, tongue movement CN XII, and smell CN I. Asymmetry may indicate facial paralysis or stroke.

Q59. Answer: B

Explanation: Cushing's triad—widened pulse pressure, bradycardia, and irregular respirations—indicates increased intracranial pressure from decreased cerebral perfusion. Normal pupils exclude acute deterioration. Bounding pulses and shallow breathing relate to cardiac or respiratory conditions, not ICP elevation.

Q60. Answer: A

Explanation: Irregular radial rhythm necessitates a one-minute apical count for accuracy and to detect possible atrial fibrillation. Short counts misrepresent irregular patterns. Peripheral pulses confirm circulation but not rhythm origin. Auscultation ensures precise cardiac evaluation.

Q61. Answer: C

Explanation: Furosemide, a loop diuretic, can cause hypokalemia and fluid loss. Monitoring potassium and daily weight identifies electrolyte imbalance and dehydration early. Apical pulse and turgor support evaluation but are secondary. Accurate tracking prevents arrhythmias and hypotension from electrolyte depletion.

Q62. Answer: C

Explanation: Hyperresonance indicates excess air, typical in emphysema due to alveolar overdistention. Pneumonia and pleural effusion cause dullness from fluid, while pulmonary edema gives crackles but not hyperresonant percussion. Assessment should include breath sounds and oxygenation for confirmation.

Q63. Answer: D

Explanation: The sequence varies—typically inspection, palpation, percussion, auscultation—except for the abdomen, where auscultation precedes palpation to avoid stimulating bowel sounds. Understanding system-specific order ensures accurate data collection without altering physiological findings.

Q64. Answer: B

Explanation: Jaundice, or yellowing of sclera, results from bilirubin accumulation due to impaired hepatic conjugation or bile flow. Carotenemia affects skin but spares sclera. Anemia causes pallor, not yellowing. Elevated bilirubin guides hepatic function evaluation.

Q65. Answer: C

Explanation: Fruity or acetone odor in breath results from ketone buildup in diabetic ketoacidosis (DKA). Uremia produces ammonia-like smell, and liver failure may cause musty odor. Recognizing characteristic breath scents assists in metabolic disorder identification and timely intervention.

Q66. Answer: B

Explanation: A pericardial friction rub is a scratchy, high-pitched sound caused by inflamed pericardial layers rubbing together, hallmark of pericarditis. It persists when patient holds breath, unlike pleural rub. Myocardial infarction causes S4 or murmurs, not rubbing.

Q67. Answer: B

Explanation: Right-sided heart failure leads to systemic venous congestion, causing jugular distension and peripheral edema. Crackles, dyspnea, and orthopnea stem from left-sided failure with pulmonary congestion. Recognizing these distinctions helps direct fluid management and diagnostic testing.

Q68. Answer: A

Explanation: Clubbing reflects long-term tissue hypoxia stimulating connective tissue proliferation at nail beds, common in COPD and cyanotic heart disease. Anemia causes pallor, not deformity. This finding warrants evaluation of oxygen saturation and chronic pulmonary status.

Q69. Answer: B

Explanation: Restoration of urine output ≥30 mL/hr reflects improved renal perfusion and overall circulatory recovery. Skin warmth and pulse strength support assessment but can vary. Diuresis confirms sustained hemodynamic stability after volume replacement.

Q70. Answer: A

Explanation: Barrel chest results from chronic overinflation in emphysema, increasing anteroposterior diameter. Muscle wasting occurs from malnutrition, not air trapping. Fluid retention or pleural effusion alters breath sounds, not chest shape. Proper positioning supports easier breathing.

Q71. Answer: B

Explanation: Hard, fixed, and non-tender nodes suggest malignancy or metastatic spread. Infections cause tender, mobile swelling. Size, texture, and mobility together distinguish benign reactive nodes from neoplastic involvement, guiding further diagnostics.

Q72. Answer: A

Explanation: Glossopharyngeal (IX) and vagus (X) nerves mediate swallowing and gag reflexes. CN VII manages facial movement, XI shoulder elevation, and XII tongue motion. Assessing reflex integrity prevents aspiration during feeding or procedures.

Q73. Answer: B

Explanation: Bowel sounds occurring more than 30 times per minute indicate hyperactivity, common with diarrhea or early obstruction. Normal activity is 5–30 per minute. Accurate timing avoids misclassification of peristaltic activity critical for gastrointestinal assessments.

Q74. Answer: A

Explanation: Stridor is a high-pitched inspiratory sound from upper airway narrowing caused by edema or obstruction. Wheezes originate from lower airway constriction. Crackles indicate alveolar fluid, and pleural rubs result from pleural friction, not obstruction. Immediate evaluation is needed.

Q75. Answer: B

Explanation: The apical pulse, auscultated over the left midclavicular fifth intercostal space, provides the most accurate measurement in infants due to small peripheral vessels. Radial or brachial pulses may be difficult to palpate and less reliable.

Q76. Answer: A

Explanation: Arterial insufficiency reduces oxygenated blood supply, producing cool, dry skin and brittle nails. Venous stasis leads to edema and brown discoloration. Dehydration affects turgor, not nail texture. Recognizing arterial signs supports early vascular management.

Q77. Answer: B

Explanation: Weber and Rinne tuning fork tests assess bone versus air conduction, distinguishing conductive from sensorineural loss. The whisper test screens acuity, not type. Snellen measures vision, and Romberg evaluates balance. Results guide audiologic referral.

Q78. Answer: A

Explanation: Cherry-red lips indicate carbon monoxide binding to hemoglobin, preventing oxygen transport despite normal SpO_2 readings. Hypoxia causes pallor or cyanosis, not redness. Immediate high-flow oxygen is necessary to displace carbon monoxide molecules.

Q79. Answer: B

Explanation: Orthostatic vitals identify postural hypotension by measuring BP and HR supine, sitting, and standing. Rapid position changes worsen symptoms. Caffeine and fluid restriction can aggravate hypotension; fluid intake and slow transitions are safer management.

Q80. Answer: C

Explanation: Accessory muscle use with cyanosis indicates severe respiratory distress and impending failure. Occasional cough and mild tachypnea are compensatory responses. Diminished bases may suggest atelectasis but not acute compromise. Immediate oxygen and provider notification are vital.

Q81. Answer: B

Explanation: Warm skin, mental alertness, and adequate urine production confirm sufficient cardiac output and tissue perfusion. Weak pulses, hypotension, or cyanosis signify inadequate perfusion. Regular assessment of these parameters ensures early detection of hemodynamic compromise.

Q82. Answer: A

Explanation: Coarse crackles result from air passing through fluid in alveoli, typical of pulmonary edema or heart failure. Bronchospasm produces wheezes, pleural thickening dampens sounds, and obstruction creates localized absence of airflow. Prompt assessment of oxygenation is essential.

Q83. Answer: B

Explanation: Classic angina or myocardial infarction presents as chest pain radiating to arm or jaw due to cardiac ischemia. Neurologic or musculoskeletal disorders cause localized pain, not radiating. Rapid ECG and cardiac enzyme evaluation are required.

Q84. Answer: A

Explanation: Normal oxygen saturation and pink nail beds signify adequate oxygen delivery. Low respiratory rate and cyanosis indicate hypoventilation or hypoxemia. Continuous SpO_2 monitoring and visual evaluation confirm oxygenation adequacy during assessment.

Q85. Answer: B

Explanation: Unequal chest movement indicates pneumothorax or pleural effusion causing lung collapse on one side. Asthma and bronchitis cause bilateral wheezing; heart failure causes crackles without asymmetry. Immediate provider notification is warranted to prevent respiratory compromise.

Q86. Answer: B

Explanation: Hemoconcentration from fluid loss elevates hematocrit levels. Bounding pulses and distension reflect fluid overload, while crackles indicate pulmonary edema. Laboratory data confirm physical findings and help guide fluid replacement therapy.

Q87. Answer: D

Explanation: Comparing bilateral pulses and checking capillary refill distinguishes systemic from localized perfusion problems. Leg elevation may worsen arterial insufficiency. Warmth and documentation alone are insufficient without thorough circulatory evaluation.

Q88. Answer: B

Explanation: The fluid wave test confirms ascites by detecting fluid movement across the abdomen when one side is tapped. Palpation alone cannot distinguish gas from fluid. Skin color assesses jaundice, while bruits evaluate vascular sounds. Documentation should include abdominal contour and girth changes.

Q89. Answer: D

Explanation: Airway and oxygenation assessment take priority in suspected stroke to prevent hypoxia-induced brain injury. Neurological checks like consciousness and grip strength follow once airway stability is ensured. Rapid recognition and activation of stroke protocol are essential.

Q90. Answer: C

Explanation: Aging reduces dermal collagen and elasticity, resulting in loose skin and fragile capillaries prone to bruising. Thickening or oil overproduction are uncommon. Understanding normal aging changes helps distinguish expected findings from pathological conditions.

Q91. Answer: B

Explanation: Pale mucous membranes and fatigue reflect reduced hemoglobin and oxygen-carrying capacity. Ruddy color occurs with polycythemia, not anemia. Bounding pulses and hypertension suggest volume overload. Assessment should include CBC to confirm anemia and evaluate severity.

Q92. Answer: B

Explanation: Wheezes result from narrowed bronchi due to bronchospasm, characteristic of asthma or COPD exacerbation. Pulmonary embolism produces sudden dyspnea, pneumonia causes crackles, and pleural effusion muffles breath sounds. Evaluate airway patency and administer prescribed bronchodilators.

Q93. Answer: C

Explanation: Dehydration concentrates blood, elevating BUN levels due to reduced renal perfusion. Low hematocrit and sodium occur with fluid overload, not deficit. Osmolality rises, not falls, as plasma becomes more concentrated. Assess hydration and renal function closely.

Q94. Answer: A

Explanation: Hypokalemia causes muscle weakness and arrhythmias due to altered cardiac conduction. Hyperreflexia and tetany occur with hypocalcemia, while hypertension and bounding pulses indicate hypervolemia. Continuous ECG monitoring is critical during electrolyte replacement therapy.

Q95. Answer: B

Explanation: A red, bulging tympanic membrane signifies acute otitis media caused by middle-ear infection and fluid accumulation. Serous otitis shows retraction with bubbles, while perforation presents with drainage. Cerumen impaction obscures visualization entirely.

Q96. Answer: B

Explanation: Brown pigmentation around ankles results from hemosiderin deposits due to chronic venous congestion. Arterial disease presents with shiny, hairless, and cool extremities. Recognizing these distinct skin changes guides accurate vascular care planning.

Q97. Answer: B

Explanation: A $PaCO_2$ of 35–45 mm Hg indicates balanced ventilation and CO_2 elimination. Normal oxygen saturation may mask hypoventilation if supplemental oxygen is used. Elevated rate and alkalosis suggest hyperventilation. Arterial blood gases provide the definitive measure.

Q98. Answer: B

Explanation: A smooth, beefy-red tongue (glossitis) indicates vitamin B_{12} deficiency causing megaloblastic anemia. Iron deficiency leads to pallor and koilonychia. Vitamins D and calcium affect bone health, not mucosal texture. Assess diet and absorption causes.

Q99. Answer: A

Explanation: Dullness over a lung base signifies fluid collection or consolidation, consistent with pleural effusion. Hyperinflation and pneumothorax yield hyperresonance. Stridor assessment applies to upper airway obstruction. Confirm findings with chest imaging for accurate diagnosis.

Q100. Answer: B

Explanation: Hypoglycemia triggers adrenergic symptoms—sweating, tremor, tachycardia, and confusion—due to low blood glucose. Polyuria and dry skin indicate hyperglycemia. Immediate carbohydrate replacement prevents neurological deterioration. Frequent glucose checks ensure early detection and stability.

Questions (101-200)

Q101. Which finding indicates left-sided heart failure?

A. Peripheral edema
B. Jugular vein distension
C. Crackles in lung bases
D. Weight gain

Q102. Which cranial nerve is assessed when testing visual fields?

A. CN II
B. CN III
C. CN IV
D. CN VI

Q103. A patient with liver disease has 3+ pitting edema. Which mechanism causes this?

A. Decreased plasma oncotic pressure
B. Increased lymphatic drainage
C. Elevated sodium intake
D. Decreased hydrostatic pressure

Q104. Which heart sound is expected in older adults due to decreased ventricular compliance?

A. S1
B. S2
C. S3
D. S4

Q105. A nurse notes a patient's respiratory pattern as deep and rapid. What term describes this?

A. Bradypnea
B. Apnea
C. Kussmaul respirations
D. Cheyne-Stokes

Q106. Which physical sign indicates chronic hypoxemia?

A. Cyanosis
B. Digital clubbing
C. Pallor
D. Diaphoresis

Q107. A nurse notes bounding pulses and moist crackles in both lungs. Which condition is likely?

A. Fluid volume deficit
B. Heart failure with volume overload
C. Hypovolemia
D. Peripheral arterial disease

Q108. Which technique ensures accurate carotid pulse assessment?

A. Palpate both arteries simultaneously
B. Palpate one side at a time
C. Use thumb pressure
D. Palpate for at least 60 seconds

Q109. What is the most appropriate action when a patient becomes short of breath during assessment?

A. Continue questioning quickly
B. Stop and allow rest with upright positioning
C. Instruct the patient to lie flat
D. Proceed with palpation

Q110. Which symptom is a classic sign of hypomagnesemia?
A. Muscle cramps and hyperactive reflexes
B. Bradycardia and lethargy
C. Hypotension with weakness
D. Drowsiness and flushing
Q111. Which clinical finding is typical of peritonitis?
A. Soft abdomen
B. Rebound tenderness
C. Hypoactive bowel sounds only
D. No guarding
Q112. A patient's tongue deviates to one side when protruded. Which cranial nerve is likely affected?
A. CN VII
B. CN X
C. CN XI
D. CN XII
Q113. Which physical assessment finding suggests dehydration in an elderly patient?
A. Slow skin recoil on sternum
B. Dry lips only
C. Bounding peripheral pulses
D. Moist oral mucosa
Q114. What does jugular venous distension primarily reflect?
A. Left atrial pressure
B. Right atrial pressure
C. Peripheral vascular resistance
D. Cardiac output
Q115. Which patient behavior is an early indicator of hypoxia?
A. Somnolence
B. Restlessness and irritability
C. Cyanosis
D. Bradycardia
Q116. During a skin assessment, the nurse notes a lesion with irregular borders and multiple colors. What is the concern?
A. Seborrheic keratosis
B. Melanoma
C. Psoriasis
D. Vitiligo
Q117. Which finding indicates effective tissue perfusion in a postoperative patient?
A. Cool extremities
B. Capillary refill <2 seconds
C. Heart rate 120 bpm
D. Systolic BP <90 mm Hg
Q118. When assessing pain, which statement reflects best nursing practice?
A. Rely on vital sign changes
B. Use the patient's self-report as the primary indicator
C. Ask family members to rate pain
D. Focus only on physical cues
Q119. A patient with COPD has an oxygen saturation of 88% on room air. What should the nurse do first?

A. Administer high-flow oxygen
B. Document as expected and continue assessment
C. Apply prescribed low-flow oxygen
D. Increase fluid intake

Q120. Which assessment tool is used to evaluate a patient's risk of pressure injury?
A. Morse Fall Scale
B. Braden Scale
C. Glasgow Coma Scale
D. Mini-Mental State Exam

Q121. Which finding suggests peripheral arterial disease (PAD)?
A. Brown pigmentation around ankles
B. Warm, red skin when legs are elevated
C. Pale, cool extremities with weak pulses
D. Soft, pitting edema

Q122. A patient reports shortness of breath when lying flat. Which term describes this symptom?
A. Orthopnea
B. Paroxysmal nocturnal dyspnea
C. Dyspnea on exertion
D. Apnea

Q123. During cardiac assessment, the nurse identifies a click following S1. What does this indicate?
A. Pericarditis
B. Mitral valve prolapse
C. Heart block
D. Aortic stenosis

Q124. Which laboratory finding is most critical to report in a patient receiving diuretic therapy?
A. Sodium 138 mEq/L
B. Potassium 2.9 mEq/L
C. Chloride 100 mEq/L
D. BUN 15 mg/dL

Q125. Which physical finding supports diagnosis of anemia?
A. Flushed face
B. Pale conjunctiva
C. Warm, moist skin
D. Increased capillary refill

Q126. What is the correct sequence for abdominal assessment?
A. Inspection, percussion, palpation, auscultation
B. Inspection, auscultation, percussion, palpation
C. Percussion, inspection, palpation, auscultation
D. Palpation, percussion, inspection, auscultation

Q127. A nurse notes pinpoint pupils bilaterally. Which condition is suspected?
A. Opioid overdose
B. Increased intracranial pressure
C. Shock
D. Alcohol intoxication

Q128. Which finding most likely indicates dehydration in a young adult?
A. Bounding pulse
B. Tachycardia and low blood pressure
C. Jugular venous distension

D. Moist mucous membranes

Q129. When assessing a wound, which drainage type indicates infection?

A. Serous

B. Sanguineous

C. Serosanguineous

D. Purulent

Q130. Which symptom suggests hypocalcemia?

A. Numbness around mouth

B. Constipation

C. Muscle flaccidity

D. Diminished reflexes

Q131. Which cardiac sound corresponds to closure of the semilunar valves?

A. S1

B. S2

C. S3

D. S4

Q132. A nurse palpates tenderness in the right lower quadrant during assessment. What condition should be suspected?

A. Appendicitis

B. Cholecystitis

C. Gastritis

D. Splenomegaly

Q133. A patient's blood pressure is 90/58 mm Hg and pulse 120 bpm. What is the most likely cause?

A. Pain response

B. Hypovolemia

C. Hypertension

D. Bradycardia

Q134. Which condition produces hyperresonant lung sounds on percussion?

A. Pleural effusion

B. Pneumothorax

C. Pneumonia

D. Atelectasis

Q135. Which finding most likely indicates renal impairment?

A. Urine output 25 mL/hr

B. Clear yellow urine 50 mL/hr

C. Urine output 1200 mL/8 hr

D. Specific gravity 1.015

Q136. During inspection, a patient's thorax expands asymmetrically with respiration. What is the likely cause?

A. Atelectasis or pneumothorax

B. Bronchitis

C. Asthma

D. Pulmonary edema

Q137. A nurse notes petechiae on a patient's lower legs. What does this suggest?

A. Normal aging

B. Capillary fragility or thrombocytopenia

C. Venous congestion

D. Allergic rash

Q138. Which finding requires immediate attention in a patient with head injury?
A. Headache
B. Vomiting once
C. Unequal pupils
D. Lethargy after sedation
Q139. A nurse notes bluish discoloration of lips and fingertips. What does this finding indicate?
A. Hyperthermia
B. Hyperoxygenation
C. Cyanosis from hypoxemia
D. Dehydration
Q140. Which neurological sign indicates increased intracranial pressure?
A. Pupils equal and reactive
B. Decerebrate posturing
C. Rapid speech
D. Hypoactive reflexes
Q141. Which abnormal heart sound is heard in early diastole and indicates heart failure?
A. S1
B. S2
C. S3
D. S4
Q142. Which laboratory test best reflects long-term glucose control?
A. Fasting blood glucose
B. Oral glucose tolerance test
C. Hemoglobin A1C
D. Serum insulin level
Q143. A nurse notes bluish discoloration of nail beds. What should be assessed next?
A. Blood pressure
B. Oxygen saturation
C. Skin turgor
D. Blood glucose
Q144. A patient reports double vision (diplopia). Which cranial nerves are involved in this function?
A. CN II, V, IX
B. CN III, IV, VI
C. CN VII, VIII, X
D. CN I, II, III
Q145. Which assessment indicates effective peripheral perfusion?
A. Capillary refill <2 seconds
B. Weak pedal pulses
C. Cool extremities
D. Delayed wound healing
Q146. Which lung sound suggests airway narrowing due to bronchospasm?
A. Crackles
B. Pleural rub
C. Wheezes
D. Stridor
Q147. A nurse observes jugular vein distension and ascites. Which condition is most consistent?
A. Left-sided heart failure
B. Right-sided heart failure

C. Pulmonary embolism
D. Hypertension

Q148. When auscultating lung fields, which sound is normal over the trachea?

A. Vesicular
B. Bronchial
C. Bronchovesicular
D. Crackles

Q149. Which cranial nerve is tested when assessing smell?

A. CN I
B. CN II
C. CN V
D. CN VII

Q150. A patient's blood pressure is 180/100 mm Hg with bounding pulses. What condition does this represent?

A. Hypovolemia
B. Hypertension
C. Heart failure
D. Dehydration

Q151. A nurse detects coarse crackles that clear after coughing. What is the likely cause?

A. Bronchitis
B. Pulmonary edema
C. Pneumothorax
D. Atelectasis

Q152. A patient exhibits 3+ deep tendon reflexes and muscle twitching. Which electrolyte imbalance should be suspected?

A. Hyperkalemia
B. Hypocalcemia
C. Hypernatremia
D. Hypomagnesemia

Q153. Which assessment finding indicates hypovolemia?

A. Flat neck veins and tachycardia
B. Bounding pulses and crackles
C. Jugular distension and edema
D. Bradycardia and hypertension

Q154. Which sign suggests increased intracranial pressure in a head-injured patient?

A. Regular respirations
B. Widening pulse pressure
C. Pinpoint pupils
D. Increased urine output

Q155. A nurse notes a patient's heart rate rises from 72 to 110 bpm after standing. What condition is suspected?

A. Orthostatic hypotension
B. Hypertension
C. Vasovagal response
D. Sinus arrhythmia

Q156. Which heart sound corresponds with closure of the atrioventricular valves?

A. S1
B. S2

C. S3
D. S4

Q157. Which characteristic finding suggests arterial ulcer rather than venous ulcer?
A. Irregular wound edges and heavy drainage
B. Pain relieved by elevation
C. Well-defined edges with minimal exudate
D. Warm surrounding skin

Q158. Which finding is consistent with metabolic acidosis?
A. Confusion and Kussmaul respirations
B. Muscle twitching and alkalosis
C. Slow, shallow breathing
D. Hypertension and bradypnea

Q159. A patient presents with tremors, anxiety, and heart rate of 120 bpm after thyroid surgery. Which condition should the nurse suspect?
A. Myxedema coma
B. Thyroid storm
C. Hypoglycemia
D. Hypocalcemia

Q160. Which sign indicates dehydration in a postoperative patient?
A. Bounding pulse
B. Dry tongue and mucous membranes
C. Crackles in lungs
D. Jugular distension

Q161. Which cardiac rhythm change is most concerning in hypokalemia?
A. Sinus bradycardia
B. Ventricular dysrhythmias
C. Sinus arrhythmia
D. Atrial fibrillation

Q162. A nurse finds a patient with unequal chest expansion and absent breath sounds on one side. What is suspected?
A. Asthma
B. Pneumothorax
C. Pneumonia
D. Bronchitis

Q163. A patient presents with severe dyspnea and pink frothy sputum. Which condition should be suspected?
A. Pulmonary embolism
B. Left-sided heart failure
C. COPD
D. Pleural effusion

Q164. Which vital sign change accompanies increased intracranial pressure (ICP)?
A. Tachycardia and hypotension
B. Bradycardia and widened pulse pressure
C. Tachypnea and hypertension
D. Rapid pulse and narrow pulse pressure

Q165. Which assessment technique is used to evaluate tactile fremitus?
A. Inspection
B. Auscultation

C. Percussion
D. Palpation

Q166. A nurse detects a bruit over the carotid artery. What does this signify?
A. Normal blood flow
B. Arterial narrowing or turbulence
C. Venous congestion
D. Heart murmur

Q167. Which finding most suggests dehydration in an adult patient?
A. Moist mucous membranes
B. Flat neck veins when supine
C. Bounding radial pulses
D. Crackles in lung bases

Q168. During inspection, scleral icterus is noted. What does this finding indicate?
A. Anemia
B. Jaundice
C. Cyanosis
D. Hypoxia

Q169. A nurse palpates a dorsalis pedis pulse rated 1+. How is this documented?
A. Absent pulse
B. Weak, thready pulse
C. Normal pulse
D. Bounding pulse

Q170. Which finding is typical of a patient with right-sided heart failure?
A. Crackles in lung bases
B. Pulmonary congestion
C. Orthopnea and dyspnea
D. Jugular vein distension and peripheral edema

Q171. When performing a neurological assessment, which finding indicates brainstem dysfunction?
A. Loss of sensation in one limb
B. Irregular respiratory pattern
C. Unilateral facial weakness
D. Memory loss

Q172. Which laboratory test is most specific for myocardial infarction?
A. CK-MB
B. Troponin I
C. Myoglobin
D. LDH

Q173. Which respiratory pattern is expected in metabolic acidosis?
A. Slow shallow respirations
B. Kussmaul respirations
C. Irregular gasping
D. Apneustic respirations

Q174. What is the primary cause of dependent edema in heart failure?
A. Dehydration
B. Venous congestion from elevated hydrostatic pressure
C. Decreased oncotic pressure
D. Increased lymphatic drainage

Q175. Which symptom indicates hyperkalemia?

A. Muscle weakness and peaked T waves
B. Hypotension and tetany
C. Paresthesia and Chvostek's sign
D. Fatigue and flattened T waves

Q176. Which assessment best evaluates peripheral circulation in the lower extremities?
A. Capillary refill and pedal pulses
B. Heart rate and rhythm
C. Respiratory pattern
D. Skin turgor

Q177. A nurse notes a patient's oxygen saturation has dropped to 86%. What should be done first?
A. Notify the physician
B. Recheck and apply oxygen per protocol
C. Check blood glucose
D. Obtain an ECG

Q178. Which sound indicates tricuspid valve closure?
A. S1
B. S2
C. S3
D. S4

Q179. A patient's BP is 80/50 mm Hg, HR 132 bpm, and skin cool and clammy. What is the priority action?
A. Administer prescribed diuretics
B. Place patient supine and elevate legs
C. Encourage deep breathing
D. Obtain urine specimen

Q180. Which finding is most concerning in a patient with COPD?
A. Barrel chest
B. Respiratory rate 10/min
C. Use of accessory muscles
D. Prolonged expiration

Q181. Which lung sound is most characteristic of pulmonary edema?
A. Wheezes
B. Coarse crackles
C. Pleural rub
D. Diminished breath sounds

Q182. A nurse notes pinpoint pupils, shallow respirations, and bradycardia. What should be suspected?
A. Opioid overdose
B. Stroke
C. Alcohol withdrawal
D. Hypoglycemia

Q183. Which assessment best confirms dehydration in an elderly patient?
A. Skin turgor on hand
B. Dry mucous membranes and concentrated urine
C. Cool extremities
D. Weight gain

Q184. Which ECG change is typical of hyperkalemia?
A. Flattened T waves

B. Peaked T waves
C. Prolonged PR interval
D. Short QT interval

Q185. A nurse palpates a vibratory sensation over the chest wall during speech. What does this represent?

A. Crepitus
B. Tactile fremitus
C. Pleural friction
D. Bronchial sound

Q186. Which finding suggests a patient may be experiencing internal bleeding post-surgery?

A. Elevated BP and bounding pulse
B. Flushed warm skin
C. Increased urine output
D. Decreased BP, tachycardia, and cool skin

Q187. A nurse notes fine tremors, restlessness, and heat intolerance. Which disorder is likely?

A. Hypothyroidism
B. Hyperthyroidism
C. Addison's disease
D. Cushing's syndrome

Q188. Which assessment tool evaluates a patient's level of consciousness?

A. Braden Scale
B. Glasgow Coma Scale
C. Morse Fall Scale
D. Mini Nutritional Assessment

Q189. Which symptom is most specific to hypocalcemia?

A. Bradycardia
B. Chvostek's sign
C. Polyuria
D. Weight gain

Q190. What is the nurse's priority when a patient suddenly develops slurred speech and right facial droop?

A. Assess blood glucose
B. Notify the stroke response team immediately
C. Check temperature
D. Review medication history

Q191. Which clinical sign indicates chronic respiratory acidosis?

A. Hyperventilation and alkalosis
B. High pH and low bicarbonate
C. Bradycardia and low CO_2
D. Confusion and elevated $PaCO_2$

Q192. Which finding suggests fluid overload?

A. Decreased jugular venous pressure
B. Crackles in lung bases
C. Poor skin turgor
D. Concentrated urine

Q193. Which heart sound is best heard at the apex using the bell of the stethoscope?

A. S1
B. S3

C. S2
D. Aortic click

Q194. A patient reports chest pain that worsens with inspiration and is relieved by leaning forward. What is suspected?
A. Myocardial infarction
B. Pericarditis
C. Pulmonary embolism
D. Aortic aneurysm

Q195. A nurse notes fruity breath odor and rapid deep respirations. Which condition is indicated?
A. Lactic acidosis
B. Diabetic ketoacidosis
C. Hypoglycemia
D. Metabolic alkalosis

Q196. Which observation indicates adequate oxygenation?
A. Cyanotic lips
B. Drowsiness
C. Restlessness
D. Warm, pink nail beds

Q197. A nurse palpates crepitus over a chest wound. What does this indicate?
A. Fluid accumulation
B. Subcutaneous emphysema
C. Pneumonia
D. Atelectasis

Q198. Which vital sign pattern suggests early shock?
A. Hypertension and bradycardia
B. Normal BP with tachycardia
C. Hypotension and bradypnea
D. Bounding pulse and fever

Q199. Which finding indicates increased intracranial pressure?
A. Tachycardia
B. Bradycardia with irregular respirations
C. Hypertension and tachypnea
D. Hypotension with rapid pulse

Q200. A nurse observes a bluish discoloration around a patient's umbilicus (Cullen's sign). What condition does this suggest?
A. Appendicitis
B. Cholecystitis
C. Peptic ulcer disease
D. Acute pancreatitis or internal bleeding

Answer key and Explanation (101-200)

Q101. Answer: C

Explanation: Crackles at lung bases occur when fluid backs into pulmonary circulation due to left ventricular failure. Right-sided failure causes peripheral edema and distension. Recognizing pulmonary congestion early enables timely diuretic therapy and oxygen support, preventing hypoxemia.

Q102. Answer: A

Explanation: Cranial nerve II, the optic nerve, transmits visual information and is assessed by checking visual acuity and peripheral fields. CN III, IV, and VI control eye movements, not vision. Impaired CN II suggests optic pathology or neurological lesion.

Q103. Answer: A

Explanation: Liver disease reduces albumin synthesis, lowering plasma oncotic pressure and allowing fluid to leak into tissues, producing edema. Increased hydrostatic pressure occurs in heart failure, while sodium excess worsens but does not initiate edema.

Q104. Answer: D

Explanation: The S4 sound occurs when atrial contraction forces blood into a stiff ventricle, common with aging or hypertension. S3 indicates fluid overload, while S1 and S2 are normal closure sounds. S4 is nonpathologic in some older adults.

Q105. Answer: C

Explanation: Kussmaul respirations are deep, rapid breaths seen in metabolic acidosis (e.g., diabetic ketoacidosis) as the body eliminates CO_2. Cheyne-Stokes alternates apnea and hyperpnea; bradypnea is slow breathing. Monitoring ABGs verifies compensation effectiveness.

Q106. Answer: B

Explanation: Clubbing—bulbous fingertip enlargement—develops from prolonged tissue hypoxia, stimulating connective tissue growth. Cyanosis signals acute hypoxia; pallor reflects anemia. Chronic respiratory disease often causes clubbing, warranting ongoing oxygen saturation monitoring.

Q107. Answer: B

Explanation: Bounding pulses and pulmonary crackles signify excess circulating volume and left-sided heart failure. Hypovolemia produces weak pulses; arterial disease causes cool extremities. Monitoring weight, urine output, and lung sounds helps gauge fluid management.

Q108. Answer: B

Explanation: Palpating one carotid artery at a time prevents vagal stimulation or cerebral perfusion compromise. Using fingertips gently is recommended; simultaneous palpation can obstruct blood flow and cause syncope.

Q109. Answer: B

Explanation: Allowing rest and placing the patient upright improves diaphragmatic expansion and gas exchange. Lying flat worsens dyspnea in respiratory compromise. Prioritize comfort and oxygen saturation assessment before resuming examination.

Q110. Answer: A

Explanation: Low magnesium increases neuromuscular excitability, causing tremors, cramps, and hyperreflexia. High magnesium produces the opposite—lethargy and depressed reflexes. Prompt replacement corrects symptoms and prevents ventricular arrhythmias associated with severe deficiency.

Q111. Answer: B

Explanation: Rebound tenderness occurs when the peritoneum is inflamed; pain intensifies upon release of pressure. It accompanies guarding and rigidity. A soft abdomen or isolated hypoactive sounds do not indicate acute peritoneal irritation. Immediate medical attention is required to prevent sepsis.

Q112. Answer: D

Explanation: Cranial nerve XII (hypoglossal) controls tongue movement. Deviation toward the affected side suggests nerve damage or stroke involvement. CN VII handles facial expression, X controls swallowing, and XI shoulder motion. Proper assessment guides neurological localization and intervention.

Q113. Answer: A

Explanation: In older adults, decreased skin elasticity makes turgor testing unreliable on the hands; the sternum gives more accuracy. Slow recoil and dry mucous membranes confirm dehydration. Bounding pulses and moist mucosa imply adequate volume or overload.

Q114. Answer: B

Explanation: Jugular venous distension indicates elevated right atrial or central venous pressure, typically from right-sided heart failure or pulmonary hypertension. It does not directly measure cardiac output or systemic resistance. Regular observation assists in fluid management.

Q115. Answer: B

Explanation: Early hypoxia causes restlessness, anxiety, and irritability as the brain senses oxygen deficit. Cyanosis and bradycardia are late, severe manifestations. Prompt oxygen assessment and airway management prevent progression to respiratory failure.

Q116. Answer: B

Explanation: Asymmetry, border irregularity, color variation, and diameter >6 mm are warning signs of malignant melanoma. Seborrheic keratosis is benign, psoriasis scaly, and vitiligo depigmented but uniform. Prompt dermatologic referral ensures early detection and treatment.

Q117. Answer: B

Explanation: Normal capillary refill under two seconds reflects adequate arterial blood flow and oxygen delivery. Tachycardia, cool skin, and hypotension signify compromised perfusion from volume loss. Continuous monitoring detects early circulatory compromise.

Q118. Answer: B

Explanation: Pain is subjective; patient self-report is the most accurate measure. Vital signs and behaviors support assessment but cannot replace personal expression. Adhering to ANA standards ensures ethical, patient-centered pain management.

Q119. Answer: C

Explanation: COPD patients often maintain baseline SpO_2 of 88–92%. Applying prescribed low-flow oxygen prevents suppressing hypoxic drive. High-flow oxygen risks CO_2 retention. Proper titration balances oxygenation and ventilation.

Q120. Answer: B

Explanation: The Braden Scale assesses risk for pressure injuries based on sensory perception, moisture, activity, mobility, nutrition, and friction/shear. Morse evaluates falls, GCS consciousness, and MMSE cognition. Early risk identification supports preventive skin care.

Q121. Answer: C

Explanation: PAD decreases arterial blood flow, producing pale, cool skin and diminished pulses. Dependent rubor appears when legs are lowered. Venous insufficiency causes brown discoloration and edema instead. Recognition of ischemic signs enables prompt vascular assessment and care.

Q122. Answer: A

Explanation: Orthopnea is difficulty breathing while supine due to pulmonary congestion from heart failure. Sitting upright relieves it. Paroxysmal nocturnal dyspnea occurs hours after sleep, while apnea means absence of breathing. Documenting severity guides management.

Q123. Answer: B

Explanation: A midsystolic click after S1 signals mitral valve prolapse caused by leaflet bulging into the atrium. Aortic stenosis produces harsh systolic murmur; pericarditis causes friction rub. Recognition aids diagnostic correlation and follow-up echocardiography.

Q124. Answer: B

Explanation: Potassium below 3.5 mEq/L increases risk of arrhythmias, especially with loop or thiazide diuretics. Sodium, chloride, and BUN are normal values. Prompt electrolyte replacement and ECG monitoring prevent cardiac complications.

Q125. Answer: B

Explanation: Pale conjunctiva reflects reduced hemoglobin and oxygenation. Flushed skin suggests polycythemia; moisture and fast refill imply adequate perfusion. Anemia evaluation requires correlating symptoms like fatigue and tachycardia with laboratory confirmation.

Q126. Answer: B

Explanation: Auscultation follows inspection to avoid stimulating peristalsis before bowel sound assessment. Percussion and palpation come afterward to determine organ size and tenderness. This sequence ensures accurate gastrointestinal findings.

Q127. Answer: A

Explanation: Opioid toxicity constricts pupils (miosis) due to central nervous system depression. ICP elevation causes unequal dilation, shock leads to dilation, and alcohol intoxication does not cause pinpoint pupils. Immediate airway and antidote assessment are vital.

Q128. Answer: B

Explanation: Tachycardia with hypotension reflects reduced circulating volume from dehydration. Bounding pulses and venous distension occur in hypervolemia. Assessing mucous membranes and urine output confirms fluid deficit and guides replacement.

Q129. Answer: D

Explanation: Purulent drainage—thick, yellow or green with odor—signals bacterial infection. Serous is clear plasma, sanguineous contains blood, and serosanguineous mixes both. Accurate documentation supports monitoring healing progression and antimicrobial effectiveness.

Q130. Answer: A

Explanation: Perioral numbness and tingling result from increased neuromuscular irritability in hypocalcemia. Constipation and weak reflexes occur in hypercalcemia. Early identification prevents tetany or cardiac dysrhythmias associated with severe calcium deficiency.

Q131. Answer: B

Explanation: S2 marks closure of the aortic and pulmonic (semilunar) valves at the end of systole. S1 corresponds to mitral and tricuspid closure. Additional heart sounds (S3, S4) reflect ventricular compliance changes, not valve closure.

Q132. Answer: A

Explanation: Right-lower-quadrant pain with rebound tenderness is classic for appendicitis due to inflammation near McBurney's point. Cholecystitis affects the right upper quadrant, gastritis the epigastric region, and splenomegaly the left upper quadrant.

Q133. Answer: B

Explanation: Low blood pressure with compensatory tachycardia indicates volume depletion or shock. Pain elevates both values but rarely lowers BP. Recognizing early hypovolemia enables prompt fluid resuscitation and hemodynamic stabilization.

Q134. Answer: B

Explanation: Pneumothorax traps air in the pleural space, causing hyperresonance from reduced tissue density. Effusion and pneumonia yield dullness due to fluid or consolidation, while atelectasis causes diminished resonance.

Q135. Answer: A

Explanation: Output below 30 mL/hr reflects reduced renal perfusion or acute kidney injury. Normal hourly output exceeds 30 mL/hr. Persistent oliguria requires evaluation of volume status and renal function tests to prevent failure progression.

Q136. Answer: A

Explanation: Unequal chest movement arises from lung collapse (atelectasis) or pneumothorax. Bronchitis and asthma produce diffuse wheezing but symmetrical expansion. Early detection of asymmetry guides imaging and chest drainage intervention.

Q137. Answer: B

Explanation: Petechiae are small, non-blanching red spots caused by capillary hemorrhage or low platelets. Venous congestion causes edema, and allergies produce pruritic rash. Investigating coagulation and platelet count is essential for diagnosis.

Q138. Answer: C

Explanation: Unequal pupils indicate increased intracranial pressure or cranial nerve III compression, requiring urgent evaluation. Headache and single vomiting episodes are common but less critical. Pupil asymmetry signals potential brain herniation risk.

Q139. Answer: C

Explanation: Cyanosis reflects low arterial oxygen saturation causing bluish skin and mucous membranes. Hyperthermia causes flushing, and dehydration leads to pallor. Assess SpO_2 and initiate oxygen therapy immediately.

Q140. Answer: B

Explanation: Decerebrate rigidity (arms extended, wrists pronated) reflects severe brainstem injury and elevated intracranial pressure. Equal pupils and normal reflexes suggest stable function. Immediate neuro intervention and monitoring are required to prevent herniation.

Q141. Answer: C

Explanation: The S3 heart sound, also called a ventricular gallop, occurs during rapid ventricular filling and signals fluid overload or left ventricular failure. It is normal in children or pregnancy but pathologic in adults, indicating decreased cardiac compliance.

Q142. Answer: C

Explanation: Hemoglobin A1C measures average blood glucose over the previous 2–3 months, reflecting glycemic control accuracy better than single tests. Fasting glucose indicates current status, and insulin levels vary widely. Monitoring A1C ensures effective diabetes management.

Q143. Answer: B

Explanation: Cyanotic nail beds indicate potential hypoxemia; checking oxygen saturation verifies arterial oxygenation status. Skin turgor and glucose are unrelated. Prompt oxygen and respiratory evaluation are vital to prevent further tissue hypoxia.

Q144. Answer: B

Explanation: Eye movements are coordinated by cranial nerves III (oculomotor), IV (trochlear), and VI (abducens). Damage causes diplopia or eye deviation. CN II mediates vision but not movement. Neurological evaluation ensures accurate localization.

Q145. Answer: A

Explanation: Rapid capillary refill suggests adequate oxygen delivery and blood flow. Weak pulses and cool extremities reflect reduced circulation, while delayed healing indicates chronic ischemia. Consistent evaluation detects early perfusion changes postoperatively.

Q146. Answer: C

Explanation: Wheezes are high-pitched musical sounds produced by airflow through constricted bronchi, common in asthma or COPD. Crackles reflect alveolar fluid; pleural rub results from pleural inflammation. Stridor indicates upper airway obstruction, not lower bronchospasm.

Q147. Answer: B

Explanation: Systemic venous congestion from right-sided heart failure causes jugular distension, hepatomegaly, and ascites. Left-sided failure leads to pulmonary symptoms. Recognizing these findings helps differentiate failure types for targeted management.

Q148. Answer: B

Explanation: Bronchial sounds—loud and high-pitched with inspiration shorter than expiration—are normal over the trachea. Vesicular sounds dominate peripheral lung fields, and bronchovesicular occur near major bronchi. Crackles indicate pathology.

Q149. Answer: A

Explanation: The olfactory nerve (CN I) mediates the sense of smell, evaluated by identifying familiar scents. CN II relates to vision, V to facial sensation, and VII to taste and expression. Loss may signal sinus disease or neurologic disorder.

Q150. Answer: B

Explanation: Elevated blood pressure and bounding pulses define hypertension due to increased systemic vascular resistance. Hypovolemia or dehydration cause low pressure and weak pulses. Continuous monitoring prevents complications such as stroke or renal damage.

Q151. Answer: A

Explanation: Crackles that resolve after coughing result from mucus in larger airways, typical of bronchitis. Pulmonary edema causes fine, persistent crackles; pneumothorax eliminates sounds unilaterally. Identifying clearing pattern distinguishes airway from alveolar pathology.

Q152. Answer: B

Explanation: Hypocalcemia increases neuromuscular excitability, producing hyperreflexia and twitching. Hyperkalemia affects cardiac rhythm, while hypernatremia causes neurologic irritability, not reflex changes. Monitoring calcium levels prevents tetany and seizures.

Q153. Answer: A

Explanation: Flat neck veins and tachycardia reflect low circulating volume. Bounding pulses and distension denote hypervolemia. Assessing BP and urine output confirms hypovolemic status for fluid replacement therapy.

Q154. Answer: B

Explanation: Widened pulse pressure accompanied by bradycardia and irregular respirations (Cushing's triad) signals elevated intracranial pressure. Pinpoint pupils arise from opioid use, and urine changes are unrelated. Prompt intervention prevents brain herniation.

Q155. Answer: A

Explanation: A significant HR increase after standing indicates orthostatic compensation for decreased venous return. It commonly accompanies volume depletion. Evaluating BP alongside HR confirms the diagnosis and guides hydration measures.

Q156. Answer: A

Explanation: S1 results from mitral and tricuspid valve closure, marking the start of systole. S2 indicates semilunar valve closure. S3 and S4 reflect ventricular filling abnormalities. Accurate identification aids cardiac auscultation interpretation.

Q157. Answer: C

Explanation: Arterial ulcers have sharply defined borders, are dry with little drainage, and result from ischemia. Venous ulcers show irregular edges and exudate. Elevation relieves venous, but worsens arterial pain due to reduced perfusion.

Q158. Answer: A

Explanation: Metabolic acidosis triggers Kussmaul respirations—deep, rapid breaths—to eliminate CO_2. Neurologic symptoms like confusion accompany acidosis. Shallow breathing or hypertension correspond to opposite imbalances. ABGs confirm the disorder.

Q159. Answer: B

Explanation: Thyroid storm is an acute hypermetabolic crisis following thyroid manipulation, presenting with tachycardia, tremor, and hyperthermia. Myxedema involves bradycardia, while hypocalcemia presents with tetany. Immediate beta-blockers and cooling measures are critical.

Q160. Answer: B

Explanation: Dry mucous membranes reflect reduced extracellular fluid volume. Bounding pulses and distension indicate overload, while crackles occur in pulmonary congestion. Monitoring intake-output ensures proper postoperative hydration management.

Q161. Answer: B

Explanation: Hypokalemia alters cardiac repolarization, increasing risk for ventricular ectopy and potentially fatal dysrhythmias like ventricular tachycardia. Bradycardia or atrial fibrillation can occur but are less specific. ECG monitoring ensures early detection and correction.

Q162. Answer: B

Explanation: Unilateral absent breath sounds and asymmetrical expansion indicate pneumothorax—air in the pleural space causing lung collapse. Pneumonia and bronchitis produce bilateral sounds; asthma causes wheezing, not absence. Immediate chest decompression may be required.

Q163. Answer: B

Explanation: Pink, frothy sputum indicates pulmonary edema secondary to left ventricular failure, where fluid backs into alveoli. Pulmonary embolism produces sudden chest pain, not frothy sputum. Prompt oxygen and diuretic therapy are essential.

Q164. Answer: B

Explanation: Cushing's triad—bradycardia, hypertension with widened pulse pressure, and irregular respirations—indicates rising ICP and brainstem compression. Early recognition prevents herniation. Regular neuro checks ensure timely intervention.

Q165. Answer: D

Explanation: Fremitus is assessed by palpation while the patient speaks ("99"); vibrations increase with consolidation and decrease with effusion or pneumothorax. It complements percussion and auscultation to identify underlying lung pathology.

Q166. Answer: B

Explanation: A bruit—whooshing sound—indicates turbulent flow from arterial stenosis or plaque. It differs from cardiac murmurs, which originate in the heart. Carotid bruits signal cerebrovascular disease risk and require further vascular imaging.

Q167. Answer: B

Explanation: Flat neck veins even when lying flat signify decreased intravascular volume. Moist mucosa and bounding pulses indicate adequate or excess volume. Crackles result from pulmonary fluid overload. Evaluate intake and urine output to confirm dehydration.

Q168. Answer: B

Explanation: Yellow sclera indicate bilirubin accumulation from hepatic dysfunction or bile obstruction. Cyanosis is bluish discoloration, anemia causes pallor, and hypoxia affects mucous membranes differently. Laboratory bilirubin testing confirms jaundice origin.

Q169. Answer: B

Explanation: A 1+ pulse is faint but palpable, described as weak or thready, suggesting decreased perfusion. 2+ is normal, 0 absent, and 3–4+ bounding. Regular comparison ensures consistent vascular assessment.

Q170. Answer: D

Explanation: Right-sided failure causes systemic venous congestion—visible jugular distension, hepatomegaly, and dependent edema. Left-sided failure leads to pulmonary congestion and crackles. Differentiation helps tailor diuretic and cardiac therapy.

Q171. Answer: B

Explanation: The brainstem regulates respiration; irregular or erratic breathing indicates dysfunction or compression. Limb weakness involves the motor cortex, and memory loss suggests cortical damage. Immediate evaluation is vital in head injury.

Q172. Answer: B

Explanation: Troponin I is the most specific and sensitive biomarker for cardiac muscle injury, rising within 3–6 hours of infarction. CK-MB is less specific, and myoglobin increases earlier but lacks cardiac exclusivity.

Q173. Answer: B

Explanation: Deep, rapid Kussmaul respirations occur as compensation for metabolic acidosis, helping eliminate excess CO_2. Shallow or irregular patterns signal inadequate compensation. Observation aids recognition of acid–base imbalance.

Q174. Answer: B

Explanation: Elevated venous hydrostatic pressure forces fluid into tissues, causing dependent edema. Reduced oncotic pressure or lymphatic obstruction also contribute but are secondary. Managing fluid volume is key to symptom control.

Q175. Answer: A

Explanation: Elevated potassium depresses cardiac conduction, producing muscle weakness and ECG peaked T waves. Hypocalcemia causes Chvostek's sign, while hypokalemia flattens T waves. Continuous cardiac monitoring ensures safety during correction.

Q176. Answer: A

Explanation: Palpating pedal pulses and checking capillary refill assess arterial blood flow to the legs. Heart rate and respiration measure systemic status but not local perfusion. Consistent findings confirm adequate circulation.

Q177. Answer: B

Explanation: Rechecking for accuracy, then applying oxygen immediately, is the correct first action for hypoxemia. Notification and ECG follow if unresponsive. Prompt intervention prevents tissue hypoxia and organ damage.

Q178. Answer: A

Explanation: The tricuspid and mitral valves close at the beginning of systole, producing the S1 sound. S2 marks closure of the aortic and pulmonic valves. Recognition ensures proper localization during cardiac auscultation.

Q179. Answer: B

Explanation: Low BP, tachycardia, and clammy skin indicate shock. Positioning the patient supine with leg elevation enhances venous return while awaiting fluid resuscitation. Immediate support prevents organ hypoperfusion.

Q180. Answer: B

Explanation: A respiratory rate of 10/min signals hypoventilation and CO_2 retention, potentially leading to respiratory failure. Barrel chest and prolonged expiration are chronic adaptations, while accessory use reflects effort but not immediate danger.

Q181. Answer: B

Explanation: Coarse crackles, especially at lung bases, indicate air passing through fluid-filled alveoli in pulmonary edema. Wheezes suggest bronchospasm, and pleural rub arises from inflammation. Recognition ensures prompt diuretic and oxygen therapy initiation.

Q182. Answer: A

Explanation: Opioid toxicity causes central nervous system depression, manifesting as miosis, slow respirations, and bradycardia. Stroke alters mental status without these signs. Immediate naloxone administration and airway support are critical interventions.

Q183. Answer: B

Explanation: Dry mucosa and dark urine accurately reflect fluid deficit. Skin elasticity decreases with aging, making turgor unreliable. Cool skin suggests vasoconstriction, not dehydration. Monitoring intake, output, and daily weight guides management.

Q184. Answer: B

Explanation: Elevated potassium shortens repolarization, producing tall, peaked T waves on ECG. Hypokalemia flattens T waves, while prolonged PR occurs with heart block. Prompt identification and treatment prevent cardiac arrest.

Q185. Answer: B

Explanation: Tactile fremitus is the palpable vibration transmitted through lung tissue during speech, increased in consolidation and decreased in pleural effusion. Crepitus indicates subcutaneous air, not vocal transmission.

Q186. Answer: D

Explanation: Hypotension, tachycardia, and cool, clammy skin signify circulatory collapse from internal bleeding. Bounding pulse and hypertension occur in overload states. Close vital monitoring and rapid surgical reporting are essential.

Q187. Answer: B

Explanation: Excess thyroid hormone increases metabolism, producing tremors, anxiety, tachycardia, and heat intolerance. Hypothyroidism shows fatigue and cold intolerance. Early detection prevents thyroid storm and cardiac strain.

Q188. Answer: B

Explanation: The Glasgow Coma Scale (GCS) objectively evaluates consciousness based on eye, verbal, and motor responses. Scores range from 3 (deep coma) to 15 (alert). Braden assesses skin risk, Morse predicts falls, and MNA evaluates nutrition. GCS is essential in head injury monitoring.

Q189. Answer: B

Explanation: Chvostek's sign—facial twitching upon tapping the facial nerve—indicates low serum calcium and neuromuscular irritability. Bradycardia and polyuria are not characteristic. Timely correction with calcium prevents tetany and cardiac dysrhythmias.

Q190. Answer: B

Explanation: Sudden neurological deficits indicate possible stroke; rapid activation of stroke protocol ensures timely imaging and thrombolytic eligibility. Delays worsen outcomes. Glucose testing follows but is not the first action.

Q191. Answer: D

Explanation: Chronic respiratory acidosis features CO_2 retention with compensatory bicarbonate elevation, often in COPD. Confusion results from carbon dioxide narcosis. Hyperventilation and high pH represent alkalosis, not acidosis.

Q192. Answer: B

Explanation: Crackles signify pulmonary congestion from fluid overload. Elevated jugular pressure and weight gain accompany it. Poor turgor and concentrated urine denote dehydration. Prompt diuretic administration helps restore fluid balance.

Q193. Answer: B

Explanation: The low-pitched S3 gallop, often signaling ventricular overload, is best heard with the bell at the apex in the left lateral position. S1 and S2 are higher-pitched and heard with the diaphragm.

Q194. Answer: B

Explanation: Pericarditis pain increases with deep breathing or lying flat and improves when leaning forward, distinguishing it from ischemic pain. A pericardial friction rub often accompanies this finding.

Q195. Answer: B

Explanation: Fruity breath and Kussmaul respirations signify diabetic ketoacidosis, where excess ketones cause acidosis. Hypoglycemia presents with sweating and tremor instead. Immediate insulin and fluid therapy correct metabolic imbalance.

Q196. Answer: D

Explanation: Pink, warm nail beds indicate sufficient arterial oxygen delivery. Cyanosis and restlessness reflect hypoxia, while drowsiness may signal CO_2 retention. Continuous SpO_2 monitoring ensures ongoing oxygen adequacy.

Q197. Answer: B

Explanation: Crepitus feels like crackling beneath the skin, caused by air escaping into subcutaneous tissue, commonly from pneumothorax or trauma. It requires monitoring for potential airway or pleural compromise.

Q198. Answer: B

Explanation: In early shock, the body maintains BP through vasoconstriction, but tachycardia signals compensation. Hypotension marks a later stage. Recognizing early indicators allows timely fluid resuscitation.

Q199. Answer: B

Explanation: Bradycardia, irregular respirations, and widened pulse pressure comprise Cushing's triad—classic for raised intracranial pressure. It indicates brainstem compression and impending herniation, requiring urgent intervention.

Q200. Answer: D

Explanation: Cullen's sign—periumbilical ecchymosis—suggests retroperitoneal bleeding, commonly from hemorrhagic pancreatitis. It indicates severe internal pathology requiring immediate diagnostic imaging and stabilization.

Questions (201-300)

Q201. Which assessment finding indicates early hypoxia?

A. Cyanosis
B. Restlessness and confusion
C. Bradycardia
D. Decreased respiratory rate

Q202. A nurse palpates the liver edge 3 cm below the costal margin. What does this suggest?

A. Normal finding
B. Hepatomegaly
C. Splenomegaly
D. Gastric distension

Q203. Which condition is indicated by positive Trousseau's sign?

A. Hyperkalemia
B. Hypocalcemia
C. Hyponatremia
D. Hypernatremia

Q204. A nurse observes a patient's hands tremor and tongue fasciculations. What should be suspected?

A. Hypoglycemia
B. Parkinson's disease
C. Hypokalemia
D. Alcohol withdrawal

Q205. Which cardiac finding occurs in pericarditis?

A. Systolic murmur
B. Friction rub
C. S3 gallop
D. Split S2

Q206. A patient with liver disease presents with confusion and asterixis. Which lab result explains this finding?

A. Low sodium
B. Elevated ammonia
C. Low albumin
D. High bilirubin

Q207. Which lung sound suggests fluid in small airways or alveoli?

A. Wheezes
B. Crackles
C. Pleural rub
D. Rhonchi

Q208. Which finding in a postoperative patient requires immediate action?

A. Mild incision pain
B. Slight nausea
C. Urine output 20 mL/hr
D. Temperature 99.8°F (37.6°C)

Q209. Which clinical sign indicates hypokalemia?

A. Muscle weakness and flattened T waves
B. Tetany and Chvostek's sign
C. Tremors and hyperreflexia

D. Peaked T waves

Q210. A nurse auscultates a high-pitched, harsh sound during inspiration over the trachea. What is this finding?

A. Wheeze
B. Stridor
C. Crackles
D. Friction rub

Q211. Which sign indicates possible meningeal irritation?

A. Positive Babinski reflex
B. Nuchal rigidity
C. Tremor
D. Flaccidity

Q212. Which test is most accurate for diagnosing deep vein thrombosis (DVT)?

A. D-dimer
B. Duplex venous ultrasound
C. Venography
D. Homan's sign

Q213. A patient with diabetes complains of tingling in the feet. What condition is suspected?

A. Peripheral neuropathy
B. Vascular occlusion
C. Electrolyte imbalance
D. Deep vein thrombosis

Q214. Which finding suggests hypoglycemia?

A. Dry skin and polyuria
B. Sweating, tremors, and confusion
C. Kussmaul respirations
D. Fruity breath odor

Q215. A nurse notes clubbing of a patient's fingers. What does this finding indicate?

A. Chronic hypoxemia
B. Dehydration
C. Hypercalcemia
D. Hyperthermia

Q216. Which symptom indicates possible hyperthyroidism?

A. Bradycardia and weight gain
B. Heat intolerance and tachycardia
C. Cold intolerance and dry skin
D. Slow speech and fatigue

Q217. Which cranial nerve is evaluated when the nurse checks gag reflex?

A. CN IX
B. CN X
C. CN XI
D. Both IX and X

Q218. A nurse observes a patient with irregularly irregular pulse rhythm. Which condition is most likely?

A. Atrial fibrillation
B. Ventricular tachycardia
C. Heart block
D. Sinus arrhythmia

Q219. Which finding is expected in fluid volume overload?
A. Hypotension and weak pulse
B. Crackles and jugular distension
C. Dry mucous membranes
D. Poor skin turgor
Q220. Which abnormal assessment finding indicates possible pneumothorax?
A. Bilateral breath sounds
B. Tracheal deviation to opposite side
C. Symmetrical chest expansion
D. Dullness to percussion
Q221. Which laboratory result supports the diagnosis of hyponatremia?
A. Serum sodium 150 mEq/L
B. Serum sodium 128 mEq/L
C. Serum potassium 4.0 mEq/L
D. Serum sodium 142 mEq/L
Q222. A patient's pupils are equal, round, and reactive to light. What does this finding indicate?
A. Brainstem injury
B. Optic nerve damage
C. Increased intracranial pressure
D. Normal neurological function
Q223. Which finding indicates a positive Babinski reflex in an adult?
A. Plantar flexion of toes
B. Dorsiflexion of great toe and fanning
C. No movement of toes
D. Rapid blinking
Q224. Which clinical manifestation is expected in hypernatremia?
A. Confusion and thirst
B. Muscle twitching and bradycardia
C. Nausea and diarrhea
D. Increased urine output with hyponatremia
Q225. A patient presents with hypotension, tachycardia, and cold clammy skin. What type of shock is suspected?
A. Cardiogenic
B. Hypovolemic
C. Septic
D. Neurogenic
Q226. Which sound is heard when the pleural surfaces become inflamed?
A. Pleural friction rub
B. Wheeze
C. Crackles
D. Rhonchi
Q227. A nurse notes a patient's skin is cool and mottled with delayed capillary refill. What does this indicate?
A. Adequate tissue perfusion
B. Peripheral vasoconstriction
C. Fluid overload
D. Elevated cardiac output
Q228. Which electrolyte imbalance is associated with positive Chvostek's and Trousseau's signs?

A. Hypokalemia
B. Hypernatremia
C. Hypocalcemia
D. Hypermagnesemia

Q229. A patient's respiratory rate is 30 breaths per minute with deep, labored breathing. What type of breathing pattern is this?
A. Cheyne-Stokes
B. Kussmaul respirations
C. Biot's respirations
D. Apneustic pattern

Q230. Which assessment finding indicates chronic arterial insufficiency?
A. Brown pigmentation
B. Dependent edema
C. Shiny, hairless legs with weak pulses
D. Warm, thickened skin

Q231. Which neurological assessment finding requires immediate intervention?
A. Pupils equal and reactive
B. New onset of unequal pupils
C. Positive gag reflex
D. Bilateral strength 5/5

Q232. Which lab finding suggests dehydration?
A. Hematocrit 52%
B. Sodium 134 mEq/L
C. BUN 10 mg/dL
D. Osmolality 275 mOsm/kg

Q233. A patient reports dizziness upon standing. What is the likely cause?
A. Orthostatic hypotension
B. Hypertension
C. Arrhythmia
D. Hypoglycemia

Q234. Which symptom is expected in a patient with hypomagnesemia?
A. Hypoactive reflexes
B. Muscle cramps and tremors
C. Lethargy
D. Bradycardia

Q235. Which clinical sign indicates fluid overload in heart failure?
A. Flat neck veins
B. Weight loss
C. Crackles and dyspnea
D. Dry mucous membranes

Q236. A patient with chronic renal failure exhibits yellow-gray skin discoloration. What causes this?
A. Carotene excess
B. Uremic pigment deposition
C. Bilirubin buildup
D. Dehydration

Q237. Which breath sound is expected over the peripheral lung fields in a healthy adult?
A. Vesicular
B. Bronchial

C. Bronchovesicular
D. Tracheal

Q238. A nurse observes slow, shallow respirations in a patient receiving morphine. What complication is this?
A. Respiratory depression
B. Hyperventilation
C. Airway obstruction
D. Bronchospasm

Q239. Which sign indicates increased central venous pressure?
A. Flat neck veins
B. Jugular venous distension
C. Weak peripheral pulses
D. Narrow pulse pressure

Q240. A patient with COPD is lethargic and has shallow respirations. What is the nurse's priority?
A. Increase oxygen flow rate immediately
B. Assess for CO_2 retention and notify provider
C. Encourage deep breathing exercises
D. Give a carbohydrate snack

Q241. Which sign indicates hypocalcemia in a postoperative thyroidectomy patient?
A. Bradycardia
B. Tingling around mouth and fingers
C. Flushed warm skin
D. Muscle flaccidity

Q242. A nurse detects an irregularly irregular pulse. Which cardiac condition is suspected?
A. Atrial fibrillation
B. Ventricular tachycardia
C. Sinus bradycardia
D. Heart block

Q243. Which finding supports the diagnosis of metabolic alkalosis?
A. Shallow respirations
B. Deep rapid breathing
C. Kussmaul respirations
D. Cyanosis

Q244. Which lab result confirms respiratory acidosis?
A. pH 7.48, $PaCO_2$ 30 mm Hg
B. pH 7.30, $PaCO_2$ 55 mm Hg
C. pH 7.50, HCO_3^- 30 mEq/L
D. pH 7.38, $PaCO_2$ 40 mm Hg

Q245. A nurse observes a patient with severe dyspnea and use of accessory muscles. What is the priority action?
A. Administer prescribed oxygen
B. Encourage coughing
C. Assess bowel sounds
D. Check blood glucose

Q246. Which condition produces dependent edema?
A. Arterial insufficiency
B. Venous congestion
C. Dehydration

D. Hypothyroidism

Q247. Which sign indicates hypovolemic shock?

A. Bounding pulse
B. Tachycardia with hypotension
C. Warm, flushed skin
D. Increased urine output

Q248. Which physical finding suggests pleural effusion?

A. Hyperresonance on percussion
B. Dullness and decreased breath sounds
C. High-pitched wheeze
D. Crackles clearing after cough

Q249. A nurse notes dry, cracked lips and poor skin turgor. Which electrolyte imbalance is suspected?

A. Hyponatremia
B. Hypernatremia
C. Hypokalemia
D. Hypocalcemia

Q250. Which cardiac sound is heard during ventricular filling and indicates volume overload?

A. S1
B. S2
C. S3
D. S4

Q251. A nurse caring for a postoperative patient notes a sudden drop in urine output. Which action should the nurse take first?

A. Notify the surgeon immediately
B. Increase IV fluid rate
C. Assess for bladder distention
D. Administer a diuretic

Q252. When implementing care for a patient with chronic heart failure, which intervention is most appropriate to evaluate effectiveness of diuretic therapy?

A. Daily weight monitoring
B. Assessing heart rate
C. Measuring oxygen saturation
D. Recording fluid intake

Q253. A nurse is developing a care plan for a patient at risk for pressure injuries. Which implementation is most effective in preventing injury?

A. Massage reddened areas every shift
B. Reposition the patient every two hours
C. Apply moisture barriers after cleansing
D. Keep heels elevated on firm surfaces

Q254. Which nursing intervention best supports effective implementation of infection control in a neutropenic patient?

A. Place the patient in airborne isolation
B. Restrict fresh flowers and unwashed fruits
C. Limit oral hygiene to once daily
D. Provide daily linen changes only if soiled

Q255. During patient education on insulin administration, which teaching strategy promotes best retention?

A. Provide written instructions only

B. Use a demonstration and return demonstration
C. Give a lecture on insulin pharmacology
D. Allow self-practice without supervision

Q256. A nurse implementing pain management for a terminally ill patient should prioritize which action?
A. Avoid opioids to prevent addiction
B. Substitute nonpharmacologic methods for drug therapy
C. Schedule analgesics only on patient request
D. Assess pain regularly and adjust medications accordingly

Q257. Which nursing intervention supports safe implementation of blood transfusion therapy?
A. Begin infusion before verifying the patient's identity
B. Use a 20-gauge catheter with normal saline
C. Add medication to the blood bag if prescribed
D. Warm the blood unit in hot water if cold

Q258. A nurse evaluating a postoperative patient's response to ambulation should report which finding to the provider?
A. Mild increase in heart rate
B. Shortness of breath and chest pain
C. Slight dizziness resolving with rest
D. Mild fatigue after walking

Q259. In planning care for a patient with COPD, which expected outcome best evaluates effective implementation?
A. Patient maintains SpO_2 of 88–92% on 2 L/min oxygen
B. Patient reports no sputum production
C. Respiratory rate stays below 12 breaths per minute
D. Lung sounds are clear bilaterally

Q260. Which intervention demonstrates proper evaluation of patient teaching about low-sodium diet adherence?
A. Ask the patient to restate sodium content recommendations
B. Recheck patient's serum sodium after one day
C. Review the patient's weekly food diary
D. Provide additional printed dietary materials

Q261. When planning discharge for a stroke patient with unilateral weakness, which collaborative action is essential?
A. Schedule follow-up only with primary care
B. Refer to physical and occupational therapy
C. Instruct family to avoid all patient activity
D. Encourage independent walking at home

Q262. The nurse implements evidence-based measures to prevent ventilator-associated pneumonia (VAP). Which action meets this standard?
A. Lower the head of the bed to 10 degrees
B. Provide oral care with chlorhexidine
C. Perform routine suctioning every hour
D. Replace ventilator tubing daily

Q263. Which step should a nurse include first when planning implementation for medication administration?
A. Verify patient allergies
B. Document the drug administration

C. Explain medication purpose to patient
D. Record vital signs afterward

Q264. During implementation of fall prevention strategies, which nursing action is most effective?
A. Place bed in high position for visibility
B. Apply side rails on all sides
C. Keep frequently used items within reach
D. Restrain the patient when alone

Q265. In evaluating wound care outcomes, which observation indicates effective implementation?
A. Drainage increases over time
B. Wound edges appear approximated and pink
C. Surrounding skin shows redness and warmth
D. Odor develops after dressing changes

Q266. Which implementation best demonstrates cultural competence in patient education?
A. Providing translated materials and verifying understanding
B. Asking the family to interpret complex medical terms
C. Teaching in English only to maintain consistency
D. Ignoring cultural beliefs that contradict treatment

Q267. A nurse implementing enteral feeding notes the patient has high gastric residuals. What should the nurse do next?
A. Continue feeding as ordered
B. Stop feeding and notify the provider
C. Decrease infusion rate by half
D. Flush with 200 mL water immediately

Q268. When implementing discharge teaching for a patient prescribed warfarin, which point is most critical?
A. Eat foods rich in vitamin K daily
B. Use a soft toothbrush and electric razor
C. Take medication at variable times
D. Double the dose if a dose is missed

Q269. Which nursing intervention ensures correct implementation of contact precautions?
A. Use sterile gloves for all care
B. Remove gloves and gown before leaving the room
C. Wear an N95 respirator during all interactions
D. Dispose of all linens in biohazard containers

Q270. When planning evaluation for a patient receiving oxygen therapy, which parameter best reflects effective treatment?
A. Capillary refill time of 4 seconds
B. Heart rate of 120 beats/minute
C. Improved alertness and stable oxygen saturation
D. Blood pressure of 150/100 mm Hg

Q271. When implementing a care plan for a patient with diabetes mellitus, which intervention should the nurse perform first before administering insulin?
A. Check the patient's current blood glucose level
B. Administer insulin with breakfast immediately
C. Instruct the patient to eat a high-protein snack
D. Review the patient's hemoglobin A1C result

Q272. A nurse evaluating a patient receiving IV antibiotics notes redness and warmth along the vein. What is the appropriate initial action?

A. Continue the infusion with a slower rate
B. Apply cold compresses to the site
C. Stop the infusion and remove the IV line
D. Flush the line with 10 mL saline

Q273. When implementing a plan for pain management, which nursing action ensures individualized care?

A. Administer analgesics on a fixed schedule regardless of pain rating
B. Evaluate pain using a standardized scale before and after interventions
C. Delay assessment to avoid disturbing the patient's rest
D. Substitute complementary methods in place of medication

Q274. Which nursing action demonstrates effective delegation during implementation?

A. Assigning sterile dressing changes to a nursing assistant
B. Delegating vital sign monitoring to an unlicensed assistive personnel
C. Instructing a student nurse to perform IV medication administration alone
D. Assigning patient teaching to a newly hired unlicensed staff member

Q275. In planning interventions for a patient with pneumonia, which implementation ensures optimal oxygenation?

A. Encourage frequent coughing and deep breathing exercises
B. Restrict oral fluids to prevent fluid overload
C. Maintain the patient in a flat supine position
D. Limit activity to complete bed rest

Q276. The nurse implementing fall precautions for an older adult with orthostatic hypotension should include which intervention?

A. Encourage rapid position changes
B. Have the patient sit briefly before standing
C. Place the bed in a high position for easier transfers
D. Remove assistive devices from reach

Q277. When implementing nutritional support for a patient with dysphagia, which action ensures safety during feeding?

A. Provide thin liquids with a straw
B. Position the patient upright at 90 degrees
C. Offer food quickly to shorten mealtime
D. Alternate solid and liquid bites rapidly

Q278. A nurse implementing a care plan for a patient with a new tracheostomy should prioritize which action?

A. Provide oral hygiene once per shift
B. Keep a spare tracheostomy tube at the bedside
C. Delay suctioning to avoid irritation
D. Use sterile saline to inflate the cuff

Q279. In implementing care for a patient receiving total parenteral nutrition (TPN), which nursing action is essential?

A. Discontinue abruptly if nausea develops
B. Use the same line for IV medications
C. Monitor blood glucose levels regularly
D. Change the TPN bag every 48 hours

Q280. When implementing postoperative respiratory care, which intervention is most effective for preventing atelectasis?

A. Encourage early ambulation and use of incentive spirometer

B. Maintain bedrest for 24 hours
C. Restrict fluids to prevent overload
D. Administer antibiotics routinely

Q281. The nurse implementing a teaching plan for a patient with new colostomy should first:
A. Assess the patient's readiness to learn
B. Demonstrate appliance change immediately
C. Provide detailed written instructions
D. Schedule follow-up in two weeks

Q282. Which implementation is most effective in preventing catheter-associated urinary tract infections (CAUTIs)?
A. Disconnect catheter tubing to obtain urine samples
B. Keep the drainage bag above bladder level
C. Maintain a closed drainage system
D. Apply antiseptic to the perineum every hour

Q283. While implementing care for a patient with hypokalemia, which action prevents complications?
A. Administer potassium IV push
B. Monitor cardiac rhythm continuously
C. Restrict dietary potassium intake
D. Encourage hyperventilation exercises

Q284. When implementing infection prevention for a patient with MRSA, which PPE sequence is correct?
A. Mask → Gown → Gloves
B. Gown → Gloves → Mask
C. Gown → Mask → Gloves
D. Gloves → Gown → Mask

Q285. A nurse evaluates effectiveness of a diabetic patient's education. Which finding indicates successful implementation?
A. The patient can list foods high in sugar
B. The patient's fasting glucose remains within target range
C. The patient asks questions about insulin types
D. The patient states diabetes is difficult to control

Q286. Which nursing action demonstrates correct implementation when administering ophthalmic drops?
A. Touch the dropper tip to the conjunctiva
B. Instill drops directly onto the cornea
C. Place drops into the conjunctival sac without touching eyelids
D. Apply drops quickly while eyes are closed

Q287. When implementing post-stroke swallowing precautions, which nursing measure is most important?
A. Allow large sips of thin liquids
B. Turn head toward unaffected side when swallowing
C. Provide small bites with chin tucked downward
D. Offer fluids through a straw

Q288. A nurse caring for a patient with peripheral IV therapy notes cool, pale skin and swelling at the site. What is the priority action?
A. Elevate the extremity and stop the infusion
B. Apply heat to promote absorption
C. Continue infusion with increased rate

D. Flush the line to restore patency
Q289. When implementing discharge education for a patient on antihypertensive therapy, which point is essential?
A. Discontinue medication once BP normalizes
B. Rise slowly from sitting or lying positions
C. Avoid monitoring BP at home
D. Double missed doses to maintain levels
Q290. When implementing enteral feeding through a nasogastric tube, what should the nurse do before starting the infusion?
A. Check for tube placement and residual volume
B. Administer feeding without delay to avoid clogging
C. Position the patient flat for comfort
D. Flush the tube only after the feeding
Q291. A nurse is implementing care for a patient with chest tubes after surgery. Which action is correct?
A. Clamp the tube during transport
B. Keep the drainage system below chest level
C. Strip the tubing every hour
D. Empty the collection chamber daily
Q292. Which nursing implementation supports effective post-operative pain management?
A. Administer analgesics only upon patient request
B. Offer scheduled analgesics before pain escalates
C. Wait for severe pain to develop before treating
D. Substitute relaxation for pharmacologic relief
Q293. When implementing a care plan for a patient with dehydration, which intervention takes priority?
A. Encourage increased oral fluid intake if alert
B. Restrict fluids until laboratory results return
C. Provide diuretics to stimulate renal function
D. Monitor weight only once daily
Q294. During implementation of a bowel training program, which nursing action is most effective?
A. Offer toileting at the same time daily
B. Increase laxative use for consistency
C. Limit fluids to reduce urgency
D. Encourage bedpan use only when necessary
Q295. Which nursing implementation best demonstrates adherence to medication safety principles?
A. Administer medication prepared by another nurse
B. Verify patient identity using two identifiers
C. Skip allergy verification if patient is stable
D. Record medication after the shift ends
Q296. When implementing care for a patient on isolation precautions, which action demonstrates correct technique?
A. Remove PPE inside the patient's room before exiting
B. Reuse gloves for multiple tasks within the same room
C. Perform hand hygiene after glove removal
D. Place used PPE on nearby surfaces for reuse
Q297. During implementation of fluid restriction for a patient with heart failure, which nursing action is appropriate?

A. Offer ice chips instead of full water glasses
B. Encourage frequent water intake to prevent dehydration
C. Hide fluids from patient to ensure compliance
D. Allow unlimited beverages if urine output is low

Q298. Which action should the nurse take first when implementing a new physician order for a high-alert medication?

A. Administer immediately to avoid delay
B. Verify dosage and order with another nurse
C. Ask patient to identify side effects
D. Document before giving the medication

Q299. When implementing care for a patient with continuous bladder irrigation, what is the nurse's primary responsibility?

A. Clamp the catheter periodically
B. Monitor urine output and color continuously
C. Replace irrigation bag every 12 hours
D. Add antibiotics to the irrigation fluid

Q300. Which intervention demonstrates correct implementation of seizure precautions?

A. Insert tongue depressor during seizure activity
B. Keep bed in low position with padded side rails
C. Restrain patient movement to prevent injury
D. Leave suction equipment outside the room

Answer key and Explanation (201-300)

Q201. Answer: B

Explanation: Early hypoxia stimulates the sympathetic system, causing restlessness, anxiety, and confusion. Cyanosis and bradycardia are late findings. Recognizing early neurobehavioral changes allows prompt oxygen and airway management before respiratory collapse develops.

Q202. Answer: B

Explanation: The liver is normally palpable only slightly below the right costal margin. Enlargement 3 cm or more indicates hepatomegaly, often from congestion or hepatitis. Splenomegaly occurs on the left, and gastric distension is central.

Q203. Answer: B

Explanation: Trousseau's sign—carpal spasm after inflating a BP cuff—indicates hypocalcemia from neuromuscular excitability. Hyperkalemia affects cardiac conduction, and sodium imbalances alter mental status rather than reflexes. Monitoring calcium prevents tetany.

Q204. Answer: D

Explanation: Fine tremors, tongue fasciculations, and agitation within 24–72 hours of alcohol cessation indicate withdrawal. Hypoglycemia causes sweating and confusion, not fasciculations. Early benzodiazepine therapy prevents seizures and delirium tremens.

Q205. Answer: B

Explanation: Pericarditis produces a friction rub—a grating, scratching sound from inflamed pericardial surfaces rubbing together. It is best heard with the diaphragm at the left sternal border. Murmurs and gallops indicate valvular or ventricular dysfunction instead.

Q206. Answer: B

Explanation: Elevated ammonia impairs cerebral function, causing hepatic encephalopathy manifested by asterixis (flapping tremor) and confusion. Bilirubin causes jaundice, while low albumin leads to edema. Reducing ammonia through lactulose improves cognition.

Q207. Answer: B

Explanation: Crackles are discontinuous popping sounds from air passing through fluid-filled alveoli, heard in pneumonia or heart failure. Wheezes indicate bronchospasm, and pleural rubs are frictional. Persistent crackles require evaluation for pulmonary edema.

Q208. Answer: C

Explanation: Urine output below 30 mL/hr indicates renal hypoperfusion or impending failure. Normal pain and mild fever are expected postoperatively. Immediate assessment of fluids and perfusion prevents irreversible kidney injury.

Q209. Answer: A

Explanation: Hypokalemia decreases cardiac excitability, producing flattened T waves and muscle weakness. Hyperreflexia and tetany arise from calcium abnormalities, while peaked T waves signify hyperkalemia. Correction prevents cardiac dysrhythmias.

Q210. Answer: B

Explanation: Stridor indicates upper airway obstruction from laryngeal edema or foreign body, producing a harsh inspiratory sound. It requires immediate airway intervention. Wheezes are expiratory and lower airway in origin.

Q211. Answer: B

Explanation: Nuchal rigidity—neck stiffness resisting flexion—is a hallmark of meningitis or meningeal irritation. Babinski is a pyramidal sign, while tremor and flaccidity suggest other neurological disorders. Early detection prevents sepsis progression.

Q212. Answer: B

Explanation: Duplex ultrasound confirms DVT by visualizing venous flow and clot presence. D-dimer supports suspicion but lacks specificity. Homan's sign is outdated and unreliable. Prompt diagnosis prevents pulmonary embolism.

Q213. Answer: A

Explanation: Tingling or burning sensations in extremities result from diabetic neuropathy due to chronic hyperglycemia damaging nerve fibers. Vascular occlusion causes pallor and pain, not tingling. Glycemic control slows progression.

Q214. Answer: B

Explanation: Hypoglycemia triggers adrenergic symptoms—sweating, tremor, and mental confusion—from low blood glucose. Polyuria and fruity breath occur in hyperglycemia. Prompt carbohydrate administration prevents neurological damage.

Q215. Answer: A

Explanation: Clubbing results from chronic tissue hypoxia stimulating soft-tissue proliferation at fingertips, seen in COPD or heart disease. It does not occur with dehydration or electrolyte imbalance. Monitoring oxygenation ensures management effectiveness.

Q216. Answer: B

Explanation: Excess thyroid hormone accelerates metabolism, causing heat intolerance, tachycardia, weight loss, and tremor. Hypothyroidism presents with fatigue and cold intolerance. Recognizing early signs prevents thyroid storm progression.

Q217. Answer: D

Explanation: Cranial nerves IX (glossopharyngeal) and X (vagus) control swallowing and gag reflex. Impairment increases aspiration risk. Assessment before oral intake ensures safe swallowing post-stroke or anesthesia.

Q218. Answer: A

Explanation: Atrial fibrillation produces an irregularly irregular rhythm due to chaotic atrial impulses. Heart block causes slow, regular rhythm, and sinus arrhythmia varies with respiration. ECG confirmation guides anticoagulant therapy.

Q219. Answer: B

Explanation: Crackles and jugular vein distension indicate pulmonary and systemic fluid overload. Weak pulses and hypotension are opposite signs of deficit. Accurate I&O tracking maintains balance and prevents heart failure exacerbation.

Q220. Answer: B

Explanation: Tracheal shift away from the affected side signals tension pneumothorax causing mediastinal displacement. Breath sounds are absent unilaterally with hyperresonance. Immediate decompression prevents respiratory collapse.

Q221. Answer: B

Explanation: Serum sodium below 135 mEq/L defines hyponatremia, which can cause confusion, muscle cramps, and seizures. Hypernatremia exceeds 145 mEq/L. Monitoring mental status and electrolytes ensures safe fluid correction.

Q222. Answer: D

Explanation: Pupils that are equal and reactive reflect intact cranial nerves II (optic) and III (oculomotor), indicating normal neurological status. Unequal or nonreactive pupils suggest brain injury or rising intracranial pressure.

Q223. Answer: B

Explanation: In adults, dorsiflexion of the big toe with fanning of others indicates a positive Babinski sign, reflecting upper motor neuron lesion. Normal adult response is plantar flexion. This sign aids neurological localization.

Q224. Answer: A

Explanation: High sodium concentration causes cellular dehydration leading to confusion, irritability, and intense thirst. Bradycardia and nausea are not typical. Monitoring neurologic status prevents complications like seizures.

Q225. Answer: B

Explanation: Hypovolemic shock results from fluid loss, producing tachycardia, hypotension, and cool, pale skin due to peripheral vasoconstriction. Septic shock presents with warm skin early; neurogenic shows bradycardia.

Q226. Answer: A

Explanation: Pleural friction rubs are coarse, grating sounds synchronous with respiration, caused by inflamed pleural membranes rubbing together. They differ from crackles, which are discontinuous and originate in alveoli.

Q227. Answer: B

Explanation: Cool, mottled skin with slow capillary refill reflects reduced peripheral perfusion due to vasoconstriction, often from shock or hypothermia. It signifies impaired oxygen delivery to tissues requiring prompt intervention.

Q228. Answer: C

Explanation: Hypocalcemia increases neuromuscular irritability, causing Chvostek's and Trousseau's signs. Hypokalemia affects cardiac conduction, while magnesium excess depresses reflexes. Prompt calcium replacement prevents tetany.

Q229. Answer: B

Explanation: Kussmaul respirations are deep and rapid, typical of metabolic acidosis as the body compensates by exhaling CO_2. Cheyne-Stokes alternates depth and apnea, and Biot's is irregular with brain injury.

Q230. Answer: C

Explanation: Arterial insufficiency causes trophic skin changes—smooth, shiny surface, hair loss, and diminished pulses due to ischemia. Venous disease presents with edema and pigmentation. Monitoring perfusion prevents ulcer formation.

Q231. Answer: B

Explanation: Sudden pupil asymmetry suggests brain herniation or intracranial pressure elevation. Equal pupils and preserved reflexes indicate normal function. Rapid physician notification is critical to prevent neurological deterioration.

Q232. Answer: A

Explanation: Elevated hematocrit reflects hemoconcentration from fluid loss. Normal BUN and osmolality argue against dehydration. Monitoring labs alongside clinical findings ensures fluid resuscitation adequacy.

Q233. Answer: A

Explanation: Orthostatic hypotension results from inadequate baroreceptor response, causing dizziness or fainting on standing due to blood pooling. Measuring BP in supine and upright positions confirms diagnosis.

Q234. Answer: B

Explanation: Low magnesium increases neuromuscular excitability, producing cramps and tremors. Hypermagnesemia causes the opposite—lethargy and decreased reflexes. Correcting magnesium prevents arrhythmias and neuromuscular dysfunction.

Q235. Answer: C

Explanation: Pulmonary crackles and dyspnea reflect excess volume backing into the lungs from left-sided heart failure. Flat veins and dryness indicate deficit. Daily weight monitoring ensures accurate volume tracking.

Q236. Answer: B

Explanation: Retained urochrome pigments in renal failure cause yellow-gray skin tint. Bilirubin buildup produces jaundice, while carotene leads to orange hue. This finding correlates with chronic uremic changes.

Q237. Answer: A

Explanation: Vesicular sounds are soft and low-pitched, heard over most lung fields, with longer inspiration than expiration. Bronchial sounds dominate over the trachea and are abnormal peripherally.

Q238. Answer: A

Explanation: Opioids suppress the medullary respiratory center, reducing rate and depth—hallmark of respiratory depression. Prompt assessment and possible naloxone administration prevent hypoventilation-induced hypoxia.

Q239. Answer: B

Explanation: Jugular distension reflects elevated central venous pressure, commonly from right-sided heart failure or volume overload. Flat veins indicate hypovolemia. CVP monitoring assists in fluid balance management.

Q240. Answer: B

Explanation: Lethargy and hypoventilation in COPD suggest CO_2 narcosis from excessive oxygen or inadequate ventilation. Oxygen titration must be cautious. Arterial blood gas evaluation confirms hypercapnia severity.

Q241. Answer: B

Explanation: Perioral and digital tingling signal hypocalcemia from accidental parathyroid removal or injury. Calcium imbalance causes neuromuscular irritability leading to tetany. Early identification allows calcium replacement to prevent seizures and laryngospasm.

Q242. Answer: A

Explanation: Atrial fibrillation produces chaotic atrial impulses, resulting in an irregularly irregular pulse. Ventricular tachycardia is fast and regular; heart block slows rhythm. Confirming with ECG is crucial for anticoagulation management.

Q243. Answer: A

Explanation: In metabolic alkalosis, hypoventilation occurs as the body retains CO_2 to compensate. Kussmaul breathing occurs in acidosis. Monitoring ABG values confirms diagnosis and guides treatment.

Q244. Answer: B

Explanation: Low pH with elevated $PaCO_2$ signifies respiratory acidosis caused by hypoventilation. The kidneys attempt compensation via bicarbonate retention. Monitoring ventilation adequacy ensures prompt correction.

Q245. Answer: A

Explanation: Accessory muscle use indicates respiratory distress and hypoxia. Administering oxygen supports gas exchange before further assessment. Delay may result in respiratory failure. Continuous SpO_2 monitoring guides titration.

Q246. Answer: B

Explanation: Venous congestion from right heart failure or prolonged standing leads to fluid accumulation in dependent areas. Arterial insufficiency causes pallor, not edema. Elevating legs aids venous return.

Q247. Answer: B

Explanation: Rapid heart rate and low blood pressure reflect compensatory response to decreased circulating volume in hypovolemic shock. Warm, flushed skin is seen in septic states. Fluid resuscitation is the immediate intervention.

Q248. Answer: B

Explanation: Pleural effusion produces dull percussion notes and diminished breath sounds due to fluid in the pleural cavity. Hyperresonance occurs in pneumothorax. Imaging confirms extent of effusion.

Q249. Answer: B
Explanation: Hypernatremia from water loss causes dehydration signs—dry mucosa, thirst, and decreased turgor. Hyponatremia leads to confusion without dryness. Adequate hydration and sodium correction are essential.
Q250. Answer: C
Explanation: The S3 gallop results from rapid ventricular filling in heart failure or fluid overload. It follows S2 and sounds like "lub-dub-ta." Early detection prevents pulmonary congestion progression.
Q251. Answer: C
Explanation: Assessing for bladder distention identifies potential urinary retention, a common postoperative complication. Jumping to interventions like fluids or diuretics may worsen the condition if obstruction exists. Immediate surgeon notification follows once the cause is verified. Critical thinking begins with assessment before intervention.
Q252. Answer: A
Explanation: Daily weights directly reflect changes in fluid status, offering early signs of diuretic effectiveness. Heart rate and oxygen levels may fluctuate for other reasons, and intake recording alone doesn't show output balance. Weight trends provide an objective and reliable measure of fluid retention control.
Q253. Answer: B
Explanation: Regular repositioning promotes circulation and relieves pressure, preventing tissue ischemia. Massaging reddened areas may worsen damage, while moisture barriers and heel supports are adjuncts, not substitutes. Scheduled position changes remain the cornerstone preventive intervention in pressure injury management.
Q254. Answer: B
Explanation: Restricting potential sources of microorganisms like plants and raw produce reduces infection risk in immunocompromised patients. Airborne isolation is unnecessary unless pathogen-specific. Limited oral hygiene increases bacterial growth, and infrequent linen changes compromise cleanliness and safety. Protective isolation principles guide all care.
Q255. Answer: B
Explanation: Demonstration with return demonstration reinforces psychomotor learning through visual and hands-on engagement. Written materials alone don't ensure comprehension, while lectures emphasize theory over skill. Supervision during practice ensures accuracy and confidence before independent administration, strengthening long-term retention and safety.
Q256. Answer: D
Explanation: Ongoing pain assessment and medication adjustment ensure comfort and dignity in end-of-life care. Addiction concerns are irrelevant in terminal settings. Waiting for requests delays relief, and nonpharmacologic measures serve as supportive, not primary, management strategies. Patient comfort remains the ethical focus.
Q257. Answer: B
Explanation: Using a 20-gauge IV with normal saline maintains patency and prevents hemolysis. Identity verification is mandatory before infusion. Medications should never mix with blood, and improper warming risks hemolysis. Following protocol ensures transfusion safety and effective circulatory support.
Q258. Answer: B
Explanation: Chest pain and dyspnea may indicate pulmonary embolism or cardiac stress, requiring immediate medical evaluation. Minor heart rate increase and transient fatigue are expected responses. Recognizing abnormal signs early prevents severe complications and promotes safe recovery progression.
Q259. Answer: A

Explanation: Maintaining appropriate oxygen saturation within prescribed limits confirms adequate gas exchange without suppressing respiratory drive. Complete absence of sputum and low respiratory rate suggest over-oxygenation. COPD management emphasizes balanced oxygen therapy and realistic outcome expectations aligned with chronic pathology.

Q260. Answer: C

Explanation: Reviewing a food diary assesses applied learning through real dietary behavior. Repetition of facts doesn't reflect lifestyle change, and serum sodium shifts take longer. Written materials support education but don't confirm adherence. Behavioral evaluation verifies true teaching effectiveness.

Q261. Answer: B

Explanation: Physical and occupational therapy maximize functional recovery, safety, and independence. Limiting activity hinders rehabilitation, and early unsupervised walking risks falls. Interdisciplinary coordination ensures comprehensive continuity of care focused on safe reintegration into home settings.

Q262. Answer: B

Explanation: Chlorhexidine oral care reduces microbial colonization, directly preventing VAP. Frequent suctioning increases mucosal trauma, and daily tubing changes are unnecessary and costly. Head elevation of 30–45 degrees complements this, maintaining best-practice standards in ventilator care implementation.

Q263. Answer: A

Explanation: Verifying allergies ensures patient safety before any medication contact. Documentation and patient teaching follow once safety is confirmed. Vital signs may guide postadministration evaluation but don't precede allergy verification. Correct sequencing prevents adverse events and reinforces nursing accountability.

Q264. Answer: C

Explanation: Keeping items within reach minimizes overreaching and unassisted movement, significantly reducing fall risk. High beds and excessive restraints increase injury potential. Proper environment arrangement supports autonomy while maintaining patient safety, aligning with nonrestrictive fall prevention protocols.

Q265. Answer: B

Explanation: Pink, approximated wound edges indicate healing and adequate perfusion. Increasing drainage, redness, and odor suggest infection or poor technique. Objective wound assessment allows evaluation of intervention effectiveness and guides ongoing modification of the care plan as needed.

Q266. Answer: A

Explanation: Using translated materials with comprehension verification ensures equitable access to information. Family interpretation risks inaccuracy and bias, while ignoring beliefs undermines trust. Cultural competence supports adherence, respect, and patient-centered outcomes across diverse healthcare populations.

Q267. Answer: B

Explanation: High residuals indicate delayed gastric emptying or intolerance; stopping feeding prevents aspiration. Adjusting rates without assessment delays care, and flushing worsens distention. Prompt provider notification ensures appropriate intervention and maintains patient safety during nutritional therapy.

Q268. Answer: B

Explanation: Using soft oral and shaving tools minimizes bleeding risk. Vitamin K intake must remain consistent, not excessive. Warfarin should be taken at the same time daily, and missed doses must not be doubled. Emphasis is on bleeding prevention and adherence consistency.

Q269. Answer: B

Explanation: Removing PPE before exiting prevents environmental contamination. Sterile gloves are unnecessary, and N95 masks apply only to airborne precautions. Linens require standard handling unless heavily soiled. Proper isolation technique safeguards both patient and staff health integrity.

Q270. Answer: C

Explanation: Improved mental status and oxygen saturation confirm adequate tissue oxygenation. Prolonged capillary refill and tachycardia indicate hypoxia, while elevated blood pressure may stem from unrelated factors. Objective and behavioral improvements validate successful oxygen therapy implementation.

Q271. Answer: A

Explanation: Blood glucose assessment ensures the correct insulin dose and prevents hypoglycemia. Administering insulin before verification can cause serious adverse effects. A1C reflects long-term control, not immediate dosing needs. Safe administration always starts with real-time glucose evaluation before medication delivery.

Q272. Answer: C

Explanation: Redness and warmth indicate phlebitis or infiltration; stopping and removing the IV prevents tissue injury. Continuing or flushing may worsen inflammation or extravasation. Cold compresses are contraindicated initially until assessment confirms the underlying cause of irritation.

Q273. Answer: B

Explanation: Using a consistent scale enables objective pain evaluation and adjustment of therapy. Fixed dosing ignores variability in pain intensity, and avoidance of assessment compromises comfort. Complementary measures are supportive but cannot replace required pharmacologic treatment when indicated.

Q274. Answer: B

Explanation: Vital signs fall within assistive personnel's role and can safely be delegated. Sterile procedures and medication administration require licensed nurse skills. Teaching patients is a professional nursing responsibility. Safe delegation matches task complexity with staff qualifications and supervision.

Q275. Answer: A

Explanation: Coughing and deep breathing enhance lung expansion, secretion clearance, and gas exchange. Restricting fluids thickens secretions, while lying flat worsens ventilation. Gradual mobilization promotes lung function recovery. Airway clearance remains the primary focus of pneumonia management.

Q276. Answer: B

Explanation: Allowing time between position changes prevents dizziness and falls. Rapid movement exacerbates hypotension, while high beds and distant devices increase risk. Gradual transitions with support maintain safety and circulation stability in vulnerable patients during mobilization.

Q277. Answer: B

Explanation: An upright position facilitates swallowing and prevents aspiration. Thin liquids and straws increase choking risk, and rapid feeding reduces airway control. Slow pacing and upright posture promote safe ingestion, especially in neurologically impaired or post-stroke patients.

Q278. Answer: B

Explanation: Having a spare tube ensures immediate replacement if accidental decannulation occurs, a potential airway emergency. Frequent oral care is important but not the highest priority. Saline is never used for cuff inflation. Airway maintenance supersedes all other interventions.

Q279. Answer: C

Explanation: Regular glucose monitoring detects hyperglycemia or hypoglycemia from TPN's high dextrose content. Abrupt discontinuation risks rebound hypoglycemia. TPN lines are exclusive and changed every 24 hours to reduce infection risk. Close glucose surveillance ensures metabolic stability.

Q280. Answer: A
Explanation: Ambulation and incentive spirometry expand alveoli, improving ventilation and preventing collapse. Bedrest delays lung recovery, and antibiotics are prophylactic only if infection risk exists. Adequate hydration supports secretion clearance and complements pulmonary hygiene measures.
Q281. Answer: A
Explanation: Assessing readiness ensures that teaching aligns with emotional and cognitive capacity. Without readiness, demonstration and written material lose effectiveness. Teaching readiness determines pacing, depth, and success of skill acquisition in major lifestyle adaptation education.
Q282. Answer: C
Explanation: A closed system prevents contamination and ascending infection. Disconnecting tubing introduces pathogens, while elevating the bag causes backflow. Excessive antiseptic use irritates tissue. Maintaining sterility and gravity drainage are central to CAUTI prevention strategies.
Q283. Answer: B
Explanation: Cardiac monitoring detects arrhythmias caused by low potassium levels. Potassium is never given IV push due to cardiac arrest risk. Restricting potassium worsens the deficit, and hyperventilation alters acid–base balance. ECG monitoring ensures safe electrolyte correction.
Q284. Answer: C
Explanation: Donning gown first prevents clothing contamination; mask protects mucous membranes, and gloves applied last maintain aseptic integrity. Proper sequence reduces transmission during patient contact. Consistent adherence reinforces both nurse and patient protection standards.
Q285. Answer: B
Explanation: Stable blood glucose demonstrates behavioral and physiological integration of education. Listing foods or expressing curiosity show partial learning but not outcome success. Objective clinical indicators confirm comprehension, adherence, and effective self-management post-teaching.
Q286. Answer: C
Explanation: Instilling drops into the conjunctival sac ensures even distribution and avoids contamination or injury. Contact with the cornea or eyelids introduces bacteria. Maintaining aseptic distance protects tissue integrity and promotes medication effectiveness in ocular therapy.
Q287. Answer: C
Explanation: Chin-tuck posture protects airway closure and facilitates safe swallowing. Thin liquids and straws increase aspiration risk. Turning toward the affected side aids pharyngeal control. Safety and aspiration prevention drive all dysphagia-related nursing interventions.
Q288. Answer: A
Explanation: These signs indicate infiltration; stopping infusion and elevating the limb prevent further tissue injury. Flushing or continuing infusion forces fluid into subcutaneous tissue. Heat is avoided unless specifically ordered. Early intervention preserves vein integrity.
Q289. Answer: B
Explanation: Gradual position changes prevent dizziness and falls caused by orthostatic hypotension, a common effect of antihypertensive drugs. Stopping medications abruptly can trigger rebound hypertension. Home monitoring encourages adherence and control. Missed doses should never be doubled for safety.
Q290. Answer: A
Explanation: Verifying placement and residual prevents aspiration and ensures gastrointestinal tolerance. Initiating feeding without confirmation risks misplacement and complications. The patient should remain upright, and flushing before and after feeding maintains patency. Safety checks always precede infusion.
Q291. Answer: B

Explanation: Gravity drainage requires positioning the system below chest level to prevent backflow. Clamping risks pneumothorax, stripping increases negative pressure, and emptying chambers compromises accuracy. Maintaining proper setup ensures effective pleural drainage and lung re-expansion.

Q292. Answer: B

Explanation: Scheduled analgesia prevents pain peaks, improving comfort and recovery. Waiting for severe pain complicates control. Nonpharmacologic methods are adjuncts, not replacements. Anticipatory management enhances mobility, breathing, and overall patient satisfaction with surgical recovery care.

Q293. Answer: A

Explanation: Encouraging oral fluids restores volume safely when the patient can swallow. Restricting intake worsens imbalance, and diuretics aggravate loss. Frequent monitoring of hydration indicators supports early correction. Rehydration is a critical intervention in dehydration management.

Q294. Answer: A

Explanation: Establishing a consistent routine promotes bowel regularity by conditioning reflexes. Laxative dependence and fluid restriction interfere with natural bowel function. Consistency and timing optimize physiological regulation and patient autonomy in long-term elimination management.

Q295. Answer: B

Explanation: Double identification confirms accurate patient matching and prevents errors. Administering others' prepared doses or skipping allergy checks violates safety standards. Immediate documentation maintains legal and clinical accuracy. Verification is a cornerstone of safe medication practice.

Q296. Answer: C

Explanation: Hand hygiene after glove removal eliminates residual pathogens, breaking the transmission chain. Removing PPE inside or reusing it increases contamination risk. Clean hands remain the single most important infection control measure in all patient care environments.

Q297. Answer: A

Explanation: Ice chips satisfy thirst with minimal volume, supporting fluid control. Excess fluid worsens heart failure symptoms, and deprivation without communication undermines trust. Education, measured portions, and accurate recording balance hydration and cardiac function effectively.

Q298. Answer: B

Explanation: Independent double-checking prevents medication errors with high-alert drugs. Immediate administration before verification risks harm, and documentation must occur afterward. Patient teaching is important but secondary to safety verification. Cross-checking ensures accuracy and compliance with institutional policy.

Q299. Answer: B

Explanation: Continuous monitoring ensures early detection of obstruction or bleeding. Clamping risks clot formation, and medication addition violates sterile protocol. Timely observation and documentation of output and color help evaluate therapy effectiveness and prevent complications post-surgery.

Q300. Answer: B

Explanation: Low bed height and padding minimize injury risk during seizures. Tongue insertion causes airway trauma, and restraints increase harm. Suction must remain available to clear secretions promptly. Proper setup anticipates events and preserves safety without restraint use.

Questions (301-400)

Q301. When implementing postoperative care for a thyroidectomy patient, which nursing action is a priority?

A. Encourage early ambulation
B. Assess for laryngeal stridor and airway obstruction
C. Provide warm fluids to soothe the throat
D. Apply a warm compress to the incision site

Q302. A nurse caring for a patient on a heparin infusion should prioritize which action?

A. Assess for signs of bleeding
B. Increase infusion rate if PTT is low
C. Stop infusion once clot dissolves
D. Flush IV with normal saline hourly

Q303. Which nursing action is most effective when implementing pressure injury prevention for an immobilized patient?

A. Apply plastic-backed sheets for cleanliness
B. Use pressure-redistributing surfaces
C. Limit repositioning to once per shift
D. Keep skin moist to prevent cracking

Q304. When implementing care for a patient receiving enteral feeding via PEG tube, which nursing intervention is correct?

A. Flush the tube with 30 mL of water before and after feeding
B. Position the patient flat for comfort
C. Administer all medications together without dilution
D. Check residual only once daily

Q305. During implementation of diabetic foot care teaching, which instruction is most appropriate?

A. Soak feet daily in hot water
B. Walk barefoot indoors to toughen skin
C. Inspect feet daily with a mirror
D. Use adhesive tape to cover blisters

Q306. When implementing care for a patient receiving IV potassium chloride, which action ensures safety?

A. Administer undiluted potassium via IV push
B. Use an infusion pump for precise control
C. Infuse rapidly to correct deficiency quickly
D. Skip cardiac monitoring during infusion

Q307. Which nursing implementation supports a safe environment for a patient with impaired vision?

A. Rearrange furniture frequently for easier access
B. Keep items and furniture in consistent locations
C. Use dim lighting to promote relaxation
D. Place call light out of reach to prevent confusion

Q308. During implementation of oxygen therapy, which nursing action prevents complications?

A. Use petroleum-based products near oxygen equipment
B. Ensure electrical equipment near oxygen is grounded
C. Remove humidification bottles to simplify setup
D. Allow smoking if flow rate is below 2 L/min

Q309. A nurse is implementing a teaching plan for a patient prescribed corticosteroids. Which instruction is essential?

A. Stop the medication once symptoms improve
B. Take the medication at bedtime
C. Do not discontinue abruptly without provider direction
D. Avoid taking the medication with food

Q310. When implementing oral care for an unconscious patient, what action ensures safety?
A. Place the patient in a supine position
B. Use large amounts of water for rinsing
C. Position the patient laterally with suction available
D. Avoid brushing teeth to prevent aspiration

Q311. Which nursing implementation is appropriate for managing a patient with a chest tube experiencing sudden absence of drainage?
A. Raise the drainage system above chest level
B. Check for kinks or dependent loops in tubing
C. Clamp the tube to prevent air entry
D. Add sterile saline to the collection chamber

Q312. During implementation of a care plan for a patient with anemia, which intervention is most effective?
A. Encourage rest periods between activities
B. Restrict dietary iron to avoid overload
C. Increase oxygen delivery only when cyanosis appears
D. Promote vigorous exercise to improve circulation

Q313. When implementing a plan of care for a patient receiving chemotherapy, which action minimizes infection risk?
A. Encourage daily raw fruit intake for vitamins
B. Avoid invasive procedures when possible
C. Group care to minimize nurse contact
D. Restrict oral hygiene to once daily

Q314. A nurse is implementing seizure safety for a patient with epilepsy. Which intervention is appropriate?
A. Place tongue depressor in the mouth during seizure
B. Turn the patient onto the side during seizure activity
C. Restrain the patient's limbs to prevent injury
D. Insert an oral airway immediately after seizure begins

Q315. When implementing postoperative care for a patient with abdominal surgery, which action prevents respiratory complications?
A. Encourage use of incentive spirometer hourly
B. Maintain strict bedrest for the first 24 hours
C. Withhold pain medication to promote alertness
D. Limit coughing to avoid incision strain

Q316. During implementation of blood transfusion therapy, what is the nurse's priority action if the patient develops chills and fever?
A. Slow the infusion rate and observe
B. Stop the transfusion immediately
C. Administer acetaminophen and continue
D. Notify the lab after transfusion completes

Q317. Which nursing action demonstrates effective implementation of skin care for a patient with incontinence?
A. Cleanse with soap and hot water after each episode

B. Apply moisture barrier cream to perineal area
C. Limit fluid intake to reduce accidents
D. Use tight-fitting briefs to absorb leakage

Q318. When implementing patient-controlled analgesia (PCA) for postoperative pain, which nursing action ensures safe use?
A. Allow family members to press the PCA button
B. Educate patient about timing and lockout function
C. Disable alarms to reduce noise
D. Administer additional opioids between PCA doses

Q319. When implementing a teaching plan for a newly diagnosed hypertensive patient, which topic should the nurse emphasize first?
A. Importance of medication adherence
B. Long-term complications of hypertension
C. Community exercise program availability
D. Dietary sodium guidelines in detail

Q320. The nurse implementing fall prevention measures in a hospital room should take which action?
A. Keep bed alarm activated and call light accessible
B. Raise all side rails at all times
C. Dim lights to promote rest
D. Move frequently used items to a high shelf

Q321. When implementing care for a patient with COPD receiving oxygen therapy, which nursing action is essential?
A. Maintain oxygen flow at prescribed low rate
B. Increase flow to 10 L/min if dyspnea occurs
C. Use a non-rebreather mask routinely
D. Encourage complete bedrest to conserve energy

Q322. During implementation of postoperative wound care, which action ensures proper sterile technique?
A. Touch sterile field edges to adjust setup
B. Keep hands above waist level during the procedure
C. Place sterile items on a moist surface
D. Reuse gloves for multiple dressings

Q323. A nurse implementing care for a patient with fluid overload should include which intervention?
A. Measure weight daily at the same time
B. Encourage increased sodium intake
C. Restrict ambulation to reduce cardiac strain
D. Discontinue diuretics when edema improves

Q324. When implementing patient education for anticoagulant therapy, which teaching is essential?
A. Avoid using soft toothbrushes
B. Report any unusual bleeding or bruising
C. Take double doses if one is missed
D. Stop medication before long flights

Q325. A nurse implementing care for a patient receiving a nasogastric suction should perform which action?
A. Maintain intermittent low suction
B. Clamp tubing continuously to preserve pressure
C. Advance the tube daily for patency
D. Instill 30 mL air every two hours

Q326. When implementing care for a patient with heart failure, which nursing action evaluates effectiveness of diuretic therapy?
A. Monitor lung sounds for decreased crackles
B. Measure heart rate only once daily
C. Encourage increased fluid intake
D. Reduce daily weight monitoring
Q327. When implementing care for a patient with a new colostomy, which nursing action is essential during appliance change?
A. Clean the stoma with alcohol pads
B. Measure stoma size each time before applying the wafer
C. Use cold water to constrict stoma vessels
D. Remove the wafer by pulling quickly
Q328. During implementation of care for a patient receiving opioids, which action is most important?
A. Assess respiratory rate and sedation level regularly
B. Withhold fluids to prevent nausea
C. Encourage rapid ambulation for bowel motility
D. Avoid using pain scales after medication
Q329. When implementing teaching for a patient on a low-cholesterol diet, which food choice demonstrates understanding?
A. Fried chicken and buttered vegetables
B. Grilled salmon with steamed broccoli
C. Sausage and scrambled eggs
D. Cheeseburger and fries
Q330. A nurse caring for a patient on contact precautions should take which action before leaving the room?
A. Remove gloves and gown before touching the door handle
B. Carry used linens to the utility room
C. Disinfect gloves with alcohol gel
D. Remove PEE after leaving the isolation area
Q331. When implementing a care plan for a patient with deep vein thrombosis (DVT), which intervention is most appropriate?
A. Massage the affected leg to promote circulation
B. Encourage early ambulation
C. Apply compression stockings as prescribed
D. Elevate legs only during sleep
Q332. During implementation of nutrition therapy for a patient with renal failure, which food should be restricted?
A. Fresh fruits
B. Processed meats
C. White bread
D. Green beans
Q333. A nurse implementing fall precautions for a confused elderly patient should include which action?
A. Place the patient near the nurses' station
B. Raise all side rails for safety
C. Remove assistive devices from reach
D. Leave bed alarm off during the day
Q334. When implementing postoperative wound irrigation, which step maintains aseptic technique?

A. Reuse the same syringe for multiple wounds
B. Direct solution flow from least to most contaminated area
C. Hold syringe 1 inch from the wound surface
D. Touch the wound edge with the syringe tip

Q335. A nurse caring for a patient with hypoglycemia should implement which immediate intervention?

A. Administer 15 g of simple carbohydrates
B. Give subcutaneous insulin
C. Increase IV fluid rate
D. Restrict oral intake

Q336. When implementing care for a patient on chemotherapy, which dietary teaching supports mucosal healing?

A. Choose spicy, coarse-textured foods
B. Use alcohol-based mouth rinses
C. Eat soft, bland, high-protein meals
D. Avoid all fruits and vegetables

Q337. During implementation of postoperative urinary retention management, which nursing intervention is appropriate?

A. Encourage the patient to void while standing or sitting upright
B. Insert a catheter immediately without assessment
C. Restrict oral fluids to avoid bladder pressure
D. Apply cold compress to the suprapubic area

Q338. When implementing a teaching plan for a patient starting anticoagulant therapy, which statement indicates understanding?

A. "I'll use an electric razor for shaving."
B. "I can take aspirin for mild pain."
C. "I should avoid wearing shoes indoors."
D. "I can skip my lab tests if I feel fine."

Q339. When applying infection control precautions for a patient with C. difficile, which intervention is most important?

A. Use alcohol-based hand sanitizer after glove removal
B. Wash hands thoroughly with soap and water
C. Wear an N95 mask for all contact
D. Reuse gowns for the same patient

Q340. A nurse implementing care for a patient with postoperative pain should take which initial step?

A. Assess pain intensity using a validated scale
B. Administer analgesics immediately
C. Encourage distraction before assessment
D. Delay intervention until provider evaluation

Q341. When implementing oxygen therapy for a COPD patient, which assessment finding requires prompt provider notification?

A. SpO_2 90% on 2 L/min oxygen
B. Drowsiness and decreased respiratory rate
C. Mild exertional dyspnea
D. Productive cough with clear sputum

Q342. When implementing preoperative teaching, which instruction best supports postoperative recovery?

A. Avoid coughing after surgery to prevent pain

B. Practice deep breathing and incentive spirometer use
C. Remain in bed until staples are removed
D. Stop ambulation until incision fully heals

Q343. During implementation of a care plan for a patient receiving digoxin, which nursing action ensures safety?

A. Administer dose if heart rate is above 50 bpm
B. Check apical pulse for one full minute before giving
C. Give dose even if patient reports visual changes
D. Skip potassium assessment before administration

Q344. When implementing care for a patient with pneumonia, which intervention promotes airway clearance?

A. Encourage fluid intake of 2–3 liters per day if tolerated
B. Limit mobility to conserve energy
C. Use antitussives routinely to reduce coughing
D. Restrict humidified oxygen

Q345. When implementing a teaching plan for insulin administration, which point must be emphasized?

A. Rotate injection sites systematically
B. Use the same site repeatedly for absorption consistency
C. Massage the injection site vigorously after injection
D. Store insulin in the freezer for stability

Q346. During implementation of tracheostomy care, which nursing action maintains airway patency?

A. Use sterile technique during suctioning
B. Instill large saline volumes before suction
C. Suction continuously for at least 30 seconds
D. Skip preoxygenation to save time

Q347. When implementing infection control for a patient with tuberculosis, which nursing action is appropriate?

A. Use a surgical mask when entering the room
B. Apply an N95 respirator before contact
C. Place the patient in a contact isolation room
D. Cohort with another respiratory patient

Q348. During implementation of IV antibiotic therapy, the nurse notes swelling and coolness at the site. What should be done first?

A. Continue the infusion slowly
B. Stop the infusion and remove the IV line
C. Apply a cold compress to the site
D. Increase the infusion rate to restore patency

Q349. A nurse implementing care for a patient with COPD should prioritize which action?

A. Encourage diaphragmatic and pursed-lip breathing
B. Administer oxygen at 6 L/min continuously
C. Encourage bedrest to minimize fatigue
D. Restrict fluid intake to reduce sputum

Q350. When implementing postoperative care for a patient after hip replacement, which action prevents dislocation?

A. Avoid using abduction pillows while in bed
B. Keep legs crossed when sitting
C. Maintain hip abduction with a wedge

D. Flex the hip beyond 90 degrees

Q351. When implementing fluid restriction in a patient with hyponatremia, which intervention supports adherence?

A. Remove all fluids from the bedside
B. Offer ice chips to relieve thirst
C. Allow unlimited fluids between meals
D. Replace fluids with caffeinated beverages

Q352. A nurse implementing safety measures for a patient at risk of seizures should:

A. Place padded side rails and suction equipment at bedside
B. Restrain patient during convulsion
C. Insert oral airway before seizure onset
D. Keep bed in high position for visibility

Q353. When implementing a teaching plan for a patient starting an iron supplement, which instruction is correct?

A. Take the supplement with milk
B. Use a straw when taking liquid iron
C. Stop medication if stools become dark
D. Take iron with antacids for comfort

Q354. When implementing post-transfusion care, which finding requires immediate action?

A. Mild fatigue after infusion
B. Shortness of breath and back pain
C. Warm sensation in the arm
D. Slight elevation in temperature

Q355. A nurse implementing postoperative teaching for a patient after abdominal surgery should include which intervention?

A. Splint incision with a pillow when coughing
B. Avoid deep breathing to reduce pain
C. Lie flat immediately after meals
D. Restrict ambulation for five days

Q356. When implementing a care plan for a patient on anticoagulants, which safety precaution is essential?

A. Use firm toothbrushes for oral hygiene
B. Report black, tarry stools promptly
C. Take double doses if a dose is missed
D. Engage in high-impact sports for exercise

Q357. When implementing post-thoracentesis care, which nursing assessment is most important?

A. Monitor for increased shortness of breath
B. Encourage oral fluid intake
C. Change dressing every two hours
D. Assist with frequent ambulation

Q358. A nurse implementing care for a patient with a nasogastric tube connected to suction should:

A. Clamp the tube between suctioning intervals
B. Maintain the tube below stomach level
C. Instill ice-cold water to clear obstructions
D. Keep patient supine for comfort

Q359. When implementing care for a patient with an indwelling urinary catheter, which measure prevents infection?

A. Empty drainage bag when half full

B. Keep collection bag below bladder level
C. Cleanse meatus once daily with soap
D. Disconnect tubing for specimen collection

Q360. When implementing care for a patient with diabetes mellitus, which nursing intervention prevents foot complications?
A. Inspect feet daily for cuts or blisters
B. Apply heating pads for warmth
C. Trim toenails deeply and rounded
D. Walk barefoot at home

Q361. When implementing care for a patient receiving tube feedings, which nursing action prevents aspiration?
A. Keep head of bed elevated at least 30 degrees
B. Stop feeding only at night
C. Check placement once daily
D. Clamp tube continuously after each bolus

Q362. When implementing preoperative patient teaching, which concept should the nurse emphasize?
A. Postoperative pain control and breathing exercises
B. Fasting ends once anesthesia starts
C. Family should leave before recovery
D. Medications can be taken the morning of surgery

Q363. When implementing care for a patient with chronic kidney disease, which dietary teaching is correct?
A. Choose processed meats for easy nutrition
B. Increase protein to promote healing
C. Encourage unlimited fluid intake
D. Limit foods high in potassium and phosphorus

Q364. A nurse implementing postoperative ambulation teaching should instruct the patient to:
A. Begin ambulation as soon as possible after surgery
B. Wait 48 hours before getting out of bed
C. Request assistance only if in pain
D. Avoid movement to protect incision

Q365. When implementing wound care for a patient with a surgical drain, which action ensures safety?
A. Maintain suction and compress reservoir before closing
B. Clamp drain to prevent fluid loss
C. Empty drain only once daily
D. Pull tubing if minimal drainage appears

Q366. When implementing care for a patient with a central venous catheter, which nursing action is appropriate?
A. Scrub the hub with antiseptic before access
B. Use tap water for dressing changes
C. Flush with air to confirm patency
D. Replace dressing only when visibly soiled

Q367. When implementing a care plan for a patient receiving hemodialysis, which nursing action is essential?
A. Measure blood pressure in the access arm
B. Assess thrill and bruit over the access site
C. Restrict all fluids before dialysis

D. Apply a tourniquet above the fistula

Q368. During implementation of post-stroke rehabilitation, which intervention supports mobility recovery?

A. Encourage use of unaffected limbs only
B. Provide passive and active range-of-motion exercises
C. Delay activity until full strength returns
D. Avoid assistive devices to promote balance

Q369. When implementing care for a patient receiving continuous enteral nutrition, which action prevents aspiration?

A. Keep head of bed elevated 30–45 degrees
B. Clamp the tube between feedings
C. Administer feeding while the patient is supine
D. Flush only at the end of the day

Q370. When implementing a care plan for a patient with peripheral edema due to heart failure, which nursing action is most appropriate?

A. Elevate the legs above heart level when resting
B. Restrict position changes to avoid dizziness
C. Encourage increased sodium intake
D. Limit use of compression stockings

Q371. When implementing postoperative care for a patient after cataract surgery, which instruction should the nurse emphasize?

A. Avoid bending or lifting heavy objects
B. Rub the operated eye to relieve itching
C. Sleep on the affected side
D. Remove protective shield after a few hours

Q372. When implementing care for a patient with neutropenia, which intervention is necessary?

A. Limit oral hygiene to once daily
B. Use only alcohol-based hand rubs
C. Provide fresh flowers and fruit for comfort
D. Place the patient in a private room

Q373. When implementing care for a patient with dehydration, which assessment finding best evaluates treatment effectiveness?

A. Moist mucous membranes and improved skin turgor
B. Increased urine specific gravity
C. Decreased blood pressure
D. Dry oral mucosa

Q374. When implementing teaching for a patient prescribed digoxin, which statement indicates correct understanding?

A. "I'll check my pulse before each dose."
B. "If I feel weak, I should take an extra tablet."
C. "I'll skip my dose if my appetite improves."
D. "I should double my dose if I miss one."

Q375. When implementing care for a patient with a pressure injury, which intervention supports healing?

A. Reposition every two hours
B. Massage reddened areas to increase circulation
C. Keep the wound dry at all times
D. Apply adhesive tape directly over the wound

Q376. When implementing discharge teaching for a patient with asthma, which instruction is essential?
A. Increase activity during acute attacks
B. Skip maintenance inhaler if asymptomatic
C. Avoid monitoring peak flow readings
D. Use the rescue inhaler for sudden wheezing
Q377. When implementing pain management for a cancer patient, which nursing action reflects the best approach?
A. Administer analgesics on a regular schedule
B. Wait until pain becomes severe before treating
C. Avoid opioids to prevent dependency
D. Use only nonpharmacologic interventions
Q378. When implementing diabetic management education, which behavior demonstrates learning?
A. The patient monitors blood glucose before meals
B. The patient skips meals to lower blood sugar
C. The patient uses expired insulin to avoid waste
D. The patient reuses disposable needles for savings
Q379. When implementing safety measures for a patient receiving oxygen, which action is correct?
A. Prohibit smoking near oxygen sources
B. Use petroleum jelly for dry lips
C. Place electrical devices near the oxygen tank
D. Store oxygen cylinders horizontally
Q380. When implementing fluid therapy for a patient with hypovolemia, which finding shows effectiveness?
A. Crackles develop in both lungs
B. Jugular veins become distended
C. Blood pressure stabilizes and urine output increases
D. Weight decreases rapidly
Q381. When implementing care for a patient receiving insulin therapy, which action prevents hypoglycemia?
A. Ensure the patient eats immediately after insulin administration
B. Administer insulin before confirming meal delivery
C. Delay meals until glucose drops
D. Double insulin dose if glucose is high
Q382. When implementing care for a patient with COPD, which position promotes effective breathing?
A. Sitting leaning slightly forward with elbows on knees
B. Lying flat in bed
C. Supine with arms elevated
D. Prone position with head turned
Q383. When implementing preoperative care, which step ensures patient safety before surgery?
A. Verify correct patient, procedure, and site
B. Leave jewelry and dentures in place
C. Administer premedication before consent
D. Skip allergy verification if not documented
Q384. When implementing care for a patient receiving blood transfusion, which step ensures correct procedure?
A. Administer over 5 minutes if stable
B. Begin infusion without crossmatch results

C. Use dextrose solution for priming line
D. Verify patient identity with another nurse before starting

Q385. When implementing care for a patient with diabetes insipidus, which action is most important?
A. Monitor urine output and specific gravity closely
B. Encourage unrestricted water intake
C. Restrict fluids to prevent overload
D. Administer insulin regularly

Q386. When implementing care for a patient with postoperative nausea and vomiting, which nursing intervention is appropriate?
A. Keep the patient NPO until symptoms resolve
B. Position the patient in side-lying position
C. Provide oral fluids immediately after emesis
D. Administer food with antiemetic medication

Q387. When implementing teaching for a patient starting antihypertensive medication, which instruction is most important?
A. Rise slowly from sitting or lying positions
B. Skip doses when feeling dizzy
C. Double doses if blood pressure remains high
D. Stop medication once blood pressure normalizes

Q388. When implementing care for a patient with a nasogastric tube to suction, which finding requires immediate action?
A. Absent bowel sounds
B. Green drainage in tubing
C. Severe abdominal distention and pain
D. Dry mucous membranes

Q389. When implementing fall prevention for an older adult with impaired mobility, which intervention is most effective?
A. Use nonskid footwear and keep pathways clear
B. Turn off hallway lights at night
C. Restrain the patient to prevent wandering
D. Remove assistive devices when unattended

Q390. When implementing care for a patient with a chest tube, which observation requires immediate intervention?
A. Continuous bubbling in the water-seal chamber
B. Fluctuation of water level during respiration
C. Small air leak after coughing
D. Drainage less than 50 mL in 8 hours

Q391. When implementing postoperative care for a patient after thyroidectomy, which item should the nurse keep at the bedside?
A. Tracheostomy set
B. Suction equipment only
C. Cardiac monitor
D. Incentive spirometer

Q392. When implementing care for a patient on chemotherapy, which measure helps prevent stomatitis?
A. Brush teeth with stiff bristles
B. Use lemon-glycerin swabs for freshness
C. Eat spicy foods to stimulate appetite

D. Rinse mouth with saline several times daily

Q393. When implementing care for a patient receiving IV potassium, which precaution is essential?

A. Use an infusion pump for administration
B. Give IV push for faster correction
C. Mix potassium with dextrose solution
D. Skip cardiac monitoring during infusion

Q394. When implementing care for a patient with hypoglycemia, which intervention is appropriate?

A. Provide orange juice or glucose tablets
B. Administer long-acting insulin
C. Restrict carbohydrates until stable
D. Delay treatment until provider arrives

Q395. When implementing infection control for a patient with hepatitis B, which precaution is necessary?

A. Use gloves when handling blood or body fluids
B. Place the patient in airborne isolation
C. Require N95 respirator for all staff
D. Use separate utensils for meals

Q396. When implementing care for a patient receiving oxygen therapy via nasal cannula, which nursing action ensures comfort and safety?

A. Use petroleum jelly for dryness
B. Secure tubing tightly around ears
C. Apply water-based lubricant to nostrils
D. Place flow meter above 10 L/min

Q397. When implementing discharge teaching for a patient with heart failure, which topic should be emphasized?

A. Weigh daily and report rapid weight gain
B. Increase sodium intake for energy
C. Limit medication use to symptom flare-ups
D. Avoid follow-up appointments if feeling well

Q398. When implementing care for a patient with urinary incontinence, which nursing action promotes skin integrity?

A. Apply moisture barrier after each cleaning
B. Use talcum powder to absorb moisture
C. Avoid cleansing after each episode
D. Keep perineal area covered with plastic pads

Q399. When implementing care for a patient with COPD, which dietary recommendation supports energy conservation?

A. Eat small, frequent, high-calorie meals
B. Drink large volumes of fluid with meals
C. Avoid snacks between meals
D. Consume low-protein foods

Q400. When implementing care for a patient with burns, which intervention prevents contractures?

A. Keep joints immobilized during healing
B. Encourage early and frequent range-of-motion exercises
C. Apply continuous moist dressings without movement
D. Delay exercise until scars form

Answer key and Explanation (301-400)

Q301. Answer: B

Explanation: Airway obstruction from edema or bleeding is life-threatening after thyroid surgery. Stridor assessment allows early intervention. Warm fluids and compresses are secondary comforts but unsafe until airway stability is confirmed. Monitoring airway patency ensures patient survival.

Q302. Answer: A

Explanation: Frequent bleeding assessment detects adverse anticoagulation effects early. Adjustments to infusion rates occur under provider direction only. Therapy continues per protocol until prescribed, and unnecessary flushing risks dosing errors. Continuous vigilance prevents life-threatening hemorrhage.

Q303. Answer: B

Explanation: Specialized support surfaces reduce pressure duration and promote tissue perfusion. Plastic materials trap heat and moisture, increasing risk. Regular turning remains essential, and skin should stay clean and dry. Equipment and routine adjustments complement each other for prevention.

Q304. Answer: A

Explanation: Flushing before and after feeding maintains patency and prevents clogging. Supine positioning promotes aspiration, and mixing medications alters absorption. Regular residual checks prevent intolerance. Consistent flushing and upright posture are critical for safe feeding administration.

Q305. Answer: C

Explanation: Daily inspection detects early ulcers or injuries, preventing infection and amputation. Hot water causes burns, and barefoot walking increases trauma. Adhesive tape tears fragile skin. Ongoing visual assessment is a cornerstone of diabetic self-care and complication prevention.

Q306. Answer: B

Explanation: Infusion pumps regulate potassium flow accurately, preventing arrhythmias. Rapid or undiluted administration is fatal. Continuous ECG monitoring tracks cardiac effects during infusion. Controlled administration and vigilant monitoring uphold critical safety standards for electrolyte therapy.

Q307. Answer: B

Explanation: Consistent item placement enhances orientation and safety for visually impaired patients. Rearranging objects or dimming light increases fall risk. The call light should remain within easy reach for emergencies. Stability and organization create an environment conducive to independence and safety.

Q308. Answer: B

Explanation: Grounding electrical devices prevents sparks in oxygen-enriched environments. Petroleum products and smoking are major fire hazards. Humidification prevents mucosal dryness, especially at higher flows. Strict adherence to safety protocols ensures both patient and environmental protection.

Q309. Answer: C

Explanation: Abrupt cessation can cause adrenal insufficiency due to suppressed cortisol production. Dosing should follow provider direction and taper gradually. Morning administration mimics natural cortisol rhythm, and taking with food minimizes gastrointestinal irritation. Adherence prevents severe withdrawal complications.

Q310. Answer: C

Explanation: Lateral positioning with suction prevents aspiration during oral hygiene. Supine posture and excessive water increase risk of fluid entering the airway. Gentle brushing maintains oral integrity and reduces infection. Safe hygiene supports overall comfort and respiratory health.

Q311. Answer: B

Explanation: Tubing obstruction may block drainage; correcting kinks restores flow. Raising the system prevents gravity drainage, and clamping risks pneumothorax. Adding fluid compromises measurement accuracy. Immediate inspection and system maintenance preserve effective chest drainage function.

Q312. Answer: A

Explanation: Rest between activities conserves oxygen and minimizes fatigue from low hemoglobin levels. Iron restriction and excessive exercise worsen symptoms. Oxygen therapy is preventive, not reactive. Balancing activity and rest optimizes patient endurance and physiologic adaptation.

Q313. Answer: B

Explanation: Reducing invasive procedures lowers pathogen exposure in immunocompromised patients. Raw produce can harbor bacteria, and infrequent hygiene promotes infection. Care clustering is for rest conservation, not infection prevention. Protective strategies prioritize asepsis and gentle procedural planning.

Q314. Answer: B

Explanation: Turning the patient on their side maintains airway patency and prevents aspiration. Inserting objects into the mouth causes trauma, and restraints increase harm. Postictal airway support follows spontaneous activity cessation. Positioning ensures protection and promotes recovery without obstruction.

Q315. Answer: A

Explanation: Incentive spirometry promotes alveolar expansion and prevents atelectasis or pneumonia. Bedrest impedes lung ventilation, while withholding analgesia reduces participation in breathing exercises. Controlled coughing supports airway clearance. Early pulmonary hygiene safeguards recovery and oxygenation.

Q316. Answer: B

Explanation: Fever and chills signal a transfusion reaction requiring immediate cessation to prevent hemolysis or shock. Continuing or slowing the infusion allows further exposure. Supportive care and provider notification follow. Prompt response preserves patient safety and prevents complications.

Q317. Answer: B

Explanation: Moisture barriers protect skin integrity by preventing irritation and breakdown from urine or stool. Harsh soap and heat damage tissue, while restricting fluids risks dehydration. Proper cleansing and protective application prevent dermatitis and infection in dependent patients.

Q318. Answer: B

Explanation: Teaching the patient about the PCA's timing and lockout promotes proper self-administration and prevents overdose. Family activation bypasses safety controls, and disabling alarms compromises monitoring. Supplemental opioids require provider approval. Education ensures autonomy and safe analgesic use.

Q319. Answer: A

Explanation: Medication adherence directly influences blood pressure control and prevents end-organ damage. Education about complications and diet follows once treatment commitment is secured. Prioritizing adherence establishes the foundation for effective long-term hypertension management and patient engagement.

Q320. Answer: A

Explanation: Bed alarms and accessible call lights ensure quick assistance, reducing fall risk. Constantly raised side rails restrict movement and may cause injury. Proper lighting and accessible items support independence while maintaining safety awareness for vulnerable patients.

Q321. Answer: A

Explanation: COPD patients rely on hypoxic drive; excessive oxygen can suppress respiration. Maintaining low prescribed flow prevents CO_2 retention. Non-rebreather masks and bedrest reduce oxygen exchange efficiency. Controlled oxygen therapy ensures safe respiratory function and gas balance.

Q322. Answer: B

Explanation: Maintaining hands above the waist preserves sterility by keeping them within the sterile zone. Touching edges or moist surfaces contaminates the field. Reusing gloves compromises infection control. Consistent sterile practice prevents wound contamination and supports healing.

Q323. Answer: A

Explanation: Daily weights track fluid status precisely, guiding treatment adjustments. Sodium restriction, not increase, is recommended. Regular movement promotes circulation, and diuretic therapy continues per provider orders. Consistent measurement ensures effective management of volume excess.

Q324. Answer: B

Explanation: Bleeding is a major anticoagulant risk, requiring prompt reporting. Hard toothbrushes and dose doubling increase hemorrhage risk, while discontinuation before travel heightens clot risk. Clear education promotes safe adherence and timely detection of adverse effects.

Q325. Answer: A

Explanation: Intermittent low suction prevents mucosal injury while maintaining drainage. Continuous suction causes gastric irritation, and advancing or instilling air without indication risks displacement. Gentle, controlled suction ensures safe decompression and prevents complications in GI management.

Q326. Answer: A

Explanation: Decreasing crackles reflects reduced pulmonary congestion and diuretic efficacy. Continuous assessment of lung sounds and daily weight confirms volume status. Fluid increase counters therapy goals. Regular monitoring validates response and guides ongoing fluid management decisions.

Q327. Answer: B

Explanation: Measuring the stoma ensures proper fit, preventing leakage and skin irritation, especially during early postoperative healing when size changes. Alcohol irritates mucosa, cold water impairs blood flow, and rough removal damages skin. Consistent assessment promotes comfort and function.

Q328. Answer: A

Explanation: Continuous respiratory and sedation assessment detects early opioid-induced depression. Adequate fluids and fiber prevent constipation, and pain scales validate therapeutic effectiveness. Early identification of adverse effects ensures safe analgesic administration and patient well-being.

Q329. Answer: B

Explanation: Grilled salmon provides lean protein and omega-3 fatty acids beneficial for cardiovascular health. Fried and processed foods elevate cholesterol and saturated fat intake. Patient education emphasizes balanced, heart-healthy food choices that reduce lipid levels and promote long-term control.

Q330. Answer: A

Explanation: PPE removal before exiting prevents environmental contamination. Carrying linens or disinfecting gloves violates infection control standards. Proper disposal inside the room followed by hand hygiene maintains barrier effectiveness and reduces transmission of pathogens between patient areas.

Q331. Answer: C

Explanation: Compression stockings improve venous return and reduce clot extension risk. Massaging dislodges clots, and ambulation is restricted initially until anticoagulation stabilizes. Elevation throughout the day supports circulation. Compression therapy and elevation are cornerstones in DVT management.

Q332. Answer: B

Explanation: Processed meats contain high sodium and phosphorus, aggravating renal dysfunction. Fresh produce and low-protein grains are safer options. Dietary education focuses on limiting potassium, phosphorus, and sodium intake to prevent electrolyte imbalance and fluid overload in renal patients.

Q333. Answer: A

Explanation: Locating the patient near staff enables quick observation and intervention. Constant side rails or inaccessible devices increase injury risk. Bed alarms should remain active at all times. Environmental proximity and supervision significantly reduce fall-related incidents.

Q334. Answer: B
Explanation: Irrigating from least to most contaminated areas prevents cross-contamination. Maintaining distance ensures adequate pressure without trauma. Reusing equipment or touching the wound breaches sterility. Sequential, aseptic irrigation promotes optimal wound cleansing and tissue healing.
Q335. Answer: A
Explanation: Rapid glucose replacement reverses hypoglycemia promptly. Insulin and fluid increases worsen the condition. Once symptoms resolve, complex carbohydrates stabilize glucose levels. Prompt recognition and response prevent neuroglycopenic complications and promote metabolic safety.
Q336. Answer: C
Explanation: Soft, bland, high-protein foods promote mucosal repair and reduce irritation from stomatitis. Spicy or rough foods aggravate inflammation, and alcohol-based rinses worsen dryness. Balanced, gentle nutrition maintains integrity of mucous membranes and supports immune recovery.
Q337. Answer: A
Explanation: Upright positioning promotes bladder relaxation and normal voiding reflexes. Catheterization follows only if noninvasive methods fail. Adequate hydration supports renal function, while cold compresses increase retention. Noninvasive encouragement remains the first-line management approach.
Q338. Answer: A
Explanation: Electric razors minimize skin cuts, reducing bleeding risk. Aspirin adds anticoagulant effects and increases danger. Protective footwear prevents injury, and regular INR testing ensures therapeutic control. Safe habits are vital for long-term anticoagulant management success.
Q339. Answer: B
Explanation: Soap and water physically remove spores resistant to alcohol sanitizers. N95 masks are unnecessary for contact pathogens. Reused gowns compromise infection control. Effective handwashing is the most reliable method to prevent transmission of C. difficile infections.
Q340. Answer: A
Explanation: Assessment establishes pain characteristics and guides appropriate intervention. Administering medication without evaluation risks under- or overtreatment. Nonpharmacologic methods complement but never replace proper assessment. Pain control begins with accurate, systematic evaluation of the patient's experience.
Q341. Answer: B
Explanation: Drowsiness with low respiratory rate indicates CO_2 retention and hypoventilation due to oxygen over-administration. Target SpO_2 in COPD is 88–92%. Exertional dyspnea and clear sputum are expected. Early recognition prevents respiratory arrest from hypoxic drive suppression.
Q342. Answer: B
Explanation: Breathing exercises improve lung expansion and prevent atelectasis. Coughing and ambulation are encouraged despite mild discomfort to enhance circulation. Extended immobility increases complication risk. Preoperative education establishes expectations and reinforces active participation in recovery.
Q343. Answer: B
Explanation: Apical pulse evaluation prevents toxicity by identifying bradycardia. Visual changes suggest toxicity and warrant withholding the dose. Hypokalemia increases digoxin sensitivity, so electrolyte checks are vital. Accurate assessment ensures therapeutic benefit without cardiac complications.
Q344. Answer: A
Explanation: Hydration thins secretions, facilitating expectoration. Immobility hinders ventilation, and suppressing cough impedes clearance. Humidified oxygen prevents dryness. Adequate fluids and movement enhance mucus mobilization and lung expansion, promoting faster respiratory recovery.

Q345. Answer: A

Explanation: Site rotation prevents lipodystrophy and ensures consistent absorption. Reusing or massaging sites alters insulin uptake, and freezing damages potency. Patient education on proper injection techniques maintains glycemic stability and injection comfort.

Q346. Answer: A

Explanation: Sterile suctioning prevents infection and obstruction. Excess saline and prolonged suctioning cause hypoxia and mucosal injury. Preoxygenation maintains oxygen saturation. Adherence to sterile, time-limited technique ensures safety and effective secretion removal.

Q347. Answer: B

Explanation: TB requires airborne precautions using an N95 respirator and a negative-pressure room. Surgical masks and contact isolation are insufficient for airborne pathogens. Cohorting increases transmission risk. Strict respiratory protection prevents airborne spread to healthcare personnel and others.

Q348. Answer: B

Explanation: Coolness and swelling suggest infiltration; stopping and removing the IV prevents tissue damage. Continuing or increasing the infusion worsens extravasation. Cold compresses may be used later depending on the medication. Immediate discontinuation ensures patient safety.

Q349. Answer: A

Explanation: Diaphragmatic and pursed-lip breathing improve ventilation and prolong exhalation, reducing air trapping. High oxygen flow depresses hypoxic drive, and bedrest decreases lung expansion. Adequate fluids thin secretions. Breathing retraining optimizes gas exchange in COPD management.

Q350. Answer: C

Explanation: Abduction wedges prevent internal rotation and dislocation of the prosthetic joint. Crossing legs or flexing beyond 90 degrees increases strain on the hip joint. Proper alignment and movement restriction support healing and prosthesis integrity.

Q351. Answer: B

Explanation: Ice chips provide moisture and comfort with minimal fluid intake, supporting compliance. Total removal fosters distress, and caffeine increases diuresis, worsening imbalance. Structured restriction with patient education ensures comfort and electrolyte correction.

Q352. Answer: A

Explanation: Padded rails and suction readiness minimize injury and maintain airway patency during seizures. Restraints and oral airways increase trauma risk. Low bed positioning further prevents falls. Prepared environment ensures safe management of seizure episodes.

Q353. Answer: B

Explanation: A straw prevents tooth staining from liquid iron. Milk and antacids reduce absorption. Dark stools are expected, not concerning. Teaching proper administration enhances effectiveness and minimizes side effects of iron therapy in anemia management.

Q354. Answer: B

Explanation: Dyspnea and back pain suggest acute hemolytic reaction requiring immediate transfusion stop and notification. Minor warmth and mild fatigue may occur normally. Early recognition and prompt response prevent hemolysis-related complications and circulatory collapse.

Q355. Answer: A

Explanation: Pillow splinting supports the incision, allowing effective coughing and deep breathing while minimizing pain. Avoiding movement delays recovery, and lying flat increases reflux risk. Teaching proper support promotes comfort and reduces pulmonary complications.

Q356. Answer: B

Explanation: Black stools indicate gastrointestinal bleeding, requiring immediate reporting. Firm toothbrushes and high-impact activities risk injury. Doubling doses increases bleeding risk. Ongoing monitoring and communication ensure early detection of adverse anticoagulation effects.

Q357. Answer: A

Explanation: Dyspnea after thoracentesis may indicate pneumothorax, demanding prompt evaluation. Dressing changes are routine but secondary. Fluids and ambulation follow stability confirmation. Continuous respiratory assessment detects complications early and safeguards lung function.

Q358. Answer: B

Explanation: Gravity drainage requires tube placement below stomach level to prevent reflux. Clamping or cold irrigation risks mucosal injury and blockage. Upright positioning aids drainage and reduces aspiration. Proper setup ensures effective decompression and patient safety.

Q359. Answer: B

Explanation: Maintaining the bag below bladder level ensures one-way flow, preventing backflow contamination. Overfilled bags cause tension, and disconnection increases infection risk. Regular perineal care with sterile collection techniques supports urinary tract health and infection prevention.

Q360. Answer: A

Explanation: Daily inspection detects early injury, preventing infection and amputation. Heating pads and barefoot walking increase burn and trauma risk. Proper hygiene and protective footwear promote safety. Preventive foot care is vital in diabetic management education.

Q361. Answer: A

Explanation: Upright positioning minimizes aspiration risk by promoting gastric emptying. Frequent placement checks and continuous elevation maintain safety. Infrequent monitoring and prolonged clamping lead to complications. Positioning remains the most effective preventive measure in enteral care.

Q362. Answer: A

Explanation: Preparing patients for postoperative exercises reduces anxiety and complications. Fasting, family visitation, and medication instructions depend on provider orders. Early education enhances cooperation, promotes lung expansion, and ensures effective pain control after surgery.

Q363. Answer: D

Explanation: Potassium and phosphorus restriction prevents hyperkalemia and mineral imbalance. Excess protein worsens azotemia, and processed foods add sodium. Tailored diet education preserves renal function and stabilizes electrolyte and fluid balance in chronic kidney disease.

Q364. Answer: A

Explanation: Early ambulation prevents venous stasis, atelectasis, and constipation. Delay or immobility increases complication risk. Controlled movement promotes circulation and recovery. Teaching emphasizes gradual, assisted mobility to restore independence safely.

Q365. Answer: A

Explanation: Compressing the reservoir restores suction, ensuring effective drainage. Clamping or infrequent emptying causes fluid accumulation and infection. Premature removal risks tissue separation. Adhering to technique maintains negative pressure and promotes wound healing.

Q366. Answer: A

Explanation: Antiseptic scrubbing before access prevents bloodstream infection. Tap water and air flushing introduce contaminants and emboli. Regular scheduled sterile dressing changes ensure asepsis. Central line care demands precise sterile technique for infection control.

Q367. Answer: B

Explanation: The presence of a thrill and bruit confirms vascular access patency. Blood pressure or tourniquet use on the access arm can cause thrombosis. Fluid restriction follows provider guidance. Ongoing monitoring prevents access complications and ensures treatment effectiveness.

Q368. Answer: B
Explanation: Range-of-motion exercises prevent contractures and support neuroplasticity during recovery. Encouraging limited movement delays progress. Assistive devices enhance safety and confidence. Rehabilitation integrates physical therapy and consistent practice to restore function gradually and safely.
Q369. Answer: A
Explanation: Head elevation reduces reflux and aspiration risk by promoting gastric emptying. Supine positioning and infrequent flushing increase complications. Consistent monitoring and positioning are key safety components of continuous feeding management.
Q370. Answer: A
Explanation: Elevating the legs promotes venous return and reduces fluid accumulation. Sodium intake worsens edema, and avoiding movement delays circulation. Compression stockings support but do not replace elevation. Elevation effectively decreases swelling and improves comfort in fluid overload.
Q371. Answer: A
Explanation: Avoiding bending or lifting prevents increased intraocular pressure and surgical site disruption. Rubbing the eye or side sleeping increases injury risk. The protective shield should remain as directed. Careful postoperative teaching preserves healing and vision recovery.
Q372. Answer: D
Explanation: A private room minimizes exposure to pathogens in immunocompromised patients. Alcohol sanitizers alone do not remove spores, and fresh produce introduces microbes. Frequent gentle hygiene reduces infection risk. Protective isolation maintains sterility and safety.
Q373. Answer: A
Explanation: Improved mucous membrane moisture and skin elasticity indicate restored hydration. High urine concentration and low blood pressure signify continued deficit. Assessment of physical hydration signs verifies effective rehydration and fluid balance correction.
Q374. Answer: A
Explanation: Checking the pulse before administration detects bradycardia, preventing toxicity. Dose adjustments without direction are unsafe. Appetite changes alone don't guide dosing. Routine monitoring ensures safety and therapeutic control with cardiac glycosides like digoxin.
Q375. Answer: A
Explanation: Repositioning promotes perfusion and reduces pressure, preventing tissue necrosis. Massaging inflamed skin worsens injury, and excessive dryness delays granulation. Protective, moist wound environments support cellular repair and minimize further breakdown risk.
Q376. Answer: D
Explanation: The rescue inhaler provides immediate bronchodilation during acute symptoms. Maintenance medication must continue consistently to prevent exacerbations. Monitoring peak flow helps detect early decline. Patient understanding of medication purpose ensures safe asthma control.
Q377. Answer: A
Explanation: Scheduled analgesia maintains consistent relief, avoiding peaks of uncontrolled pain. Waiting for severe pain complicates control. Opioid dependency is not a concern in terminal care. Comprehensive management combines pharmacologic and supportive comfort measures.
Q378. Answer: A
Explanation: Regular premeal glucose checks ensure correct dosing and glycemic control. Skipping meals or reusing equipment causes instability and infection risk. Proper technique and monitoring improve safety and adherence in diabetes self-management.
Q379. Answer: A

Explanation: Oxygen supports combustion; strict no-smoking policies prevent fires. Petroleum products and improper cylinder storage increase hazards. Non-petroleum moisturizers should be used. Safety compliance prevents oxygen-related injuries and environmental accidents.

Q380. Answer: C

Explanation: Stable vital signs and improved urine output indicate restored volume. Distention and crackles reflect overload, and weight loss suggests dehydration. Ongoing evaluation ensures fluid replacement remains balanced and therapeutic without causing pulmonary congestion.

Q381. Answer: A

Explanation: Coordinating insulin with food intake prevents glucose drops. Administering insulin without available food or doubling doses risks severe hypoglycemia. Patient education on timing and symptoms strengthens safety and glycemic control practices.

Q382. Answer: A

Explanation: The tripod position facilitates diaphragm descent and accessory muscle use, easing exhalation. Supine and prone positions restrict lung expansion. Encouraging upright leaning improves oxygenation and comfort in COPD respiratory management.

Q383. Answer: A

Explanation: Surgical verification prevents wrong-site errors and meets safety protocol standards. Jewelry and dentures must be removed to prevent aspiration and electrical burns. Consent precedes medication, and allergy confirmation avoids intraoperative reactions. Verification is mandatory preoperatively.

Q384. Answer: D

Explanation: Two-nurse verification ensures compatibility and patient safety. Crossmatch confirmation and normal saline are required before infusion. Rapid administration causes volume overload. Following verification protocols prevents transfusion-related errors and adverse reactions.

Q385. Answer: A

Explanation: Excess urine output and dilute urine signal ineffective ADH activity. Monitoring output guides therapy effectiveness. Overhydration is possible but managed through balance, not restriction. Insulin is unrelated. Close tracking prevents dehydration and electrolyte imbalance.

Q386. Answer: B

Explanation: Side-lying positioning prevents aspiration and maintains airway patency during vomiting. NPO status follows until control is achieved. Immediate fluids or food aggravate nausea. Safety positioning takes priority in managing postoperative gastrointestinal discomfort.

Q387. Answer: A

Explanation: Slow positional changes prevent orthostatic hypotension, a common side effect. Skipping or doubling doses disrupts blood pressure control and increases risk for rebound hypertension. Ongoing adherence and gradual movement ensure patient safety and effective long-term management.

Q388. Answer: C

Explanation: Abdominal distention with pain may indicate obstruction or tube malfunction. Normal drainage appears greenish from bile, and mild dryness is expected. Immediate tube assessment and provider notification prevent perforation or aspiration complications during decompression therapy.

Q389. Answer: A

Explanation: Proper footwear and clear pathways minimize slipping and tripping hazards. Darkness and restraints increase injury risk and anxiety. Keeping assistive devices nearby promotes independence and safety. Environmental control and support optimize fall prevention outcomes.

Q390. Answer: A

Explanation: Continuous bubbling indicates an air leak that compromises lung re-expansion. Fluctuation is expected, and minimal drainage may occur naturally. Early recognition and correction of leaks prevent pneumothorax recurrence and ensure effective negative pressure maintenance.

Q391. Answer: A
Explanation: Airway obstruction from swelling or bleeding requires immediate tracheostomy access. Suction and oxygen follow, but a trach set provides emergency airway management. Airway protection remains the highest priority after thyroid surgery due to proximity to vital structures.
Q392. Answer: D
Explanation: Saline rinses cleanse gently without irritation and prevent mucositis. Acidic swabs and spicy foods worsen inflammation. Soft-bristle brushes protect fragile tissues. Regular saline care maintains oral hygiene and comfort during cytotoxic therapy.
Q393. Answer: A
Explanation: Infusion pumps regulate potassium flow precisely, preventing arrhythmias and overdose. Potassium must never be given as an IV push. Dextrose alters serum potassium shifts, and cardiac monitoring ensures immediate detection of adverse reactions during therapy.
Q394. Answer: A
Explanation: Quick carbohydrate intake restores glucose balance rapidly. Insulin or delays exacerbate symptoms, and carbohydrate restriction worsens hypoglycemia. Immediate response ensures brain glucose supply and prevents seizures or loss of consciousness in diabetic emergencies.
Q395. Answer: A
Explanation: Hepatitis B spreads through blood exposure, requiring standard precautions with gloves for fluid contact. Airborne isolation and respirators are unnecessary. Proper PPE and sharps handling prevent transmission effectively in healthcare environments.
Q396. Answer: C
Explanation: Water-based lubricants prevent mucosal irritation without fire risk. Petroleum products are flammable in oxygen-rich settings. Loose, properly fitted tubing avoids skin breakdown. Comfort and safety practices enhance adherence to long-term oxygen therapy.
Q397. Answer: A
Explanation: Daily weight gain signals fluid retention and worsening heart failure, requiring prompt reporting. Sodium restriction and medication adherence prevent exacerbations. Regular follow-up maintains stability and early detection of decompensation. Patient self-monitoring is essential for control.
Q398. Answer: A
Explanation: Barrier creams protect skin from moisture and breakdown. Talcum powder cakes and irritates tissue, while plastic pads trap heat and promote bacterial growth. Regular gentle cleansing with barrier application maintains comfort and prevents dermatitis.
Q399. Answer: A
Explanation: Small, high-calorie meals prevent fatigue and meet metabolic demands with minimal effort. Excess fluids during meals cause fullness and limit intake. Adequate protein preserves muscle function. Nutritional adjustments support energy balance in chronic pulmonary disease.
Q400. Answer: B
Explanation: Early mobilization maintains flexibility and prevents joint contractures. Prolonged immobility causes stiffness and functional loss. Movement within tolerance promotes circulation, reduces edema, and optimizes long-term recovery outcomes for burn survivors.

Questions (401-500)

Q401. When implementing postoperative care for a patient after abdominal surgery, which finding requires immediate action?

A. Rigid, distended abdomen and severe pain
B. Bowel sounds returning after 24 hours
C. Passing small amounts of flatus
D. Moderate incisional tenderness

Q402. When implementing care for a patient with dehydration due to vomiting, which IV fluid is most appropriate initially?

A. Normal saline (0.9% NaCl)
B. Dextrose 10% in water
C. 5% dextrose in 0.45% saline
D. Lactated Ringer's after 24 hours only

Q403. When implementing postoperative education for a patient after mastectomy, which instruction is correct?

A. Perform hand and arm exercises on the affected side
B. Avoid using the arm on the surgical side
C. Apply tight elastic bandages
D. Restrict fluid intake until drains removed

Q404. When implementing infection control in a healthcare setting, which practice is fundamental?

A. Disinfect hands with alcohol only if visibly soiled
B. Wear gloves at all times in the unit
C. Reuse gowns for the same patient
D. Perform hand hygiene before and after patient contact

Q405. When implementing care for a patient with chronic pain, which nursing approach is most therapeutic?

A. Validate the patient's pain experience
B. Focus only on objective findings
C. Encourage tolerance without intervention
D. Limit medication discussions

Q406. When implementing care for a patient with pneumonia, which nursing intervention supports airway clearance?

A. Encourage coughing and deep breathing exercises
B. Restrict fluids to prevent congestion
C. Maintain strict bed rest
D. Use sedatives to suppress cough

Q407. When implementing care for a patient with acute pancreatitis, which nursing intervention is appropriate?

A. Maintain the patient NPO with IV fluids as prescribed
B. Encourage early oral intake to promote healing
C. Administer high-fat meals to restore nutrition
D. Apply warm compresses to the abdomen

Q408. When implementing care for a patient with hypokalemia, which food choice should the nurse encourage?

A. Cottage cheese and pears
B. White rice and applesauce
C. Toast and jelly

D. Baked potatoes and bananas

Q409. When implementing teaching for a patient with a new ileostomy, which statement shows correct understanding?

A. "I'll empty the pouch when it's one-third full."
B. "I'll use alcohol to clean around the stoma."
C. "I'll avoid increasing my fluid intake."
D. "I can reuse pouches for up to a week."

Q410. When implementing postoperative care for a patient after spinal surgery, which intervention prevents complications?

A. Logroll the patient when repositioning
B. Assist the patient to sit up without support
C. Elevate the head of the bed 60 degrees
D. Encourage twisting movements for flexibility

Q411. When implementing care for a patient with hypocalcemia, which action is most appropriate?

A. Limit intake of dairy products
B. Encourage high-phosphorus foods
C. Administer loop diuretics as needed
D. Implement seizure precautions

Q412. When implementing care for a patient receiving total parenteral nutrition (TPN), which nursing intervention ensures safety?

A. Monitor blood glucose levels regularly
B. Discontinue TPN abruptly if stable
C. Hang the solution for 48 hours
D. Flush the line with saline between infusions

Q413. When implementing teaching for a patient on corticosteroid therapy, which instruction is correct?

A. Taper the dose gradually before stopping
B. Take the medication on an empty stomach
C. Stop medication immediately if symptoms resolve
D. Avoid reporting mood changes to the provider

Q414. When implementing care for a patient with a tracheostomy, which action prevents infection?

A. Use sterile technique when suctioning
B. Clean the inner cannula with tap water
C. Change ties daily without assistance
D. Avoid humidification of inspired air

Q415. When implementing care for a patient receiving IV antibiotics, which assessment finding indicates a possible allergic reaction?

A. Slight fatigue during infusion
B. Mild nausea after administration
C. Transient warmth at injection site
D. Rash and difficulty breathing

Q416. When implementing care for a patient post–total knee replacement, which intervention prevents deep vein thrombosis (DVT)?

A. Encourage use of sequential compression devices
B. Maintain bedrest for 48 hours
C. Limit fluid intake to prevent swelling
D. Avoid leg exercises to protect incision

Q417. When implementing care for a patient with a chest tube after surgery, which nursing action ensures proper function?
A. Keep the drainage system below chest level
B. Clamp the tube routinely to check patency
C. Empty the collection chamber daily
D. Strip the tubing frequently to promote flow
Q418. When implementing care for a patient receiving opioid analgesics, which nursing action prevents respiratory depression?
A. Monitor respiratory rate and sedation level frequently
B. Administer extra doses when pain persists
C. Keep naloxone at bedside but use only for cardiac arrest
D. Encourage concurrent sedative use for comfort
Q419. When implementing a teaching plan for a patient with hypertension, which instruction supports blood pressure control?
A. Limit potassium-rich foods completely
B. Avoid taking medication during weekends
C. Reduce sodium intake and exercise regularly
D. Increase processed food consumption
Q420. When implementing care for a patient on mechanical ventilation, which nursing action promotes airway safety?
A. Keep the head of the bed elevated 30–45 degrees
B. Turn off alarms during suctioning
C. Instill saline routinely before suctioning
D. Restrain all extremities continuously
Q421. When implementing postoperative teaching for a patient after coronary artery bypass grafting (CABG), which advice is appropriate?
A. Report new or increased chest pain immediately
B. Resume heavy lifting after one week
C. Avoid use of prescribed cardiac medications
D. Expect persistent low-grade fever for several weeks
Q422. When implementing care for a patient receiving enteral feeding through a PEG tube, which step ensures correct administration?
A. Verify tube placement before each feeding
B. Mix medications with the feeding solution
C. Flush the tube only once daily
D. Administer feedings with the patient supine
Q423. When implementing care for a patient with hypernatremia, which intervention is most important?
A. Restrict hypotonic IV fluids
B. Increase sodium-rich foods
C. Administer hypertonic saline
D. Encourage oral water intake if possible
Q424. When implementing care for a patient with a newly inserted Foley catheter, which nursing action is essential?
A. Secure catheter tubing to the thigh
B. Keep drainage bag above bladder level
C. Disconnect tubing for ambulation
D. Flush catheter routinely with saline

Q425. When implementing care for a patient with increased intracranial pressure (ICP), which nursing intervention is appropriate?
A. Maintain head of bed at 30 degrees
B. Encourage frequent coughing and straining
C. Keep neck flexed to promote drainage
D. Administer hypotonic IV fluids
Q426. When implementing postoperative care for a patient after abdominal surgery, which intervention promotes bowel function recovery?
A. Encourage early ambulation and fluid intake
B. Withhold all oral intake for three days
C. Avoid movement to protect sutures
D. Limit use of incentive spirometer
Q427. When implementing postoperative care for a patient after cholecystectomy, which nursing action promotes recovery?
A. Limit fluid intake to reduce nausea
B. Maintain the patient on complete bedrest
C. Encourage early ambulation to promote bile flow
D. Delay oral intake for one week
Q428. When implementing care for a patient with pneumonia, which nursing intervention aids secretion clearance?
A. Encourage frequent coughing and deep breathing
B. Limit fluid intake to prevent fluid overload
C. Encourage shallow breathing to reduce pain
D. Maintain the patient in a supine position
Q429. When implementing care for a patient receiving diuretics, which assessment finding requires immediate action?
A. Irregular heart rate and muscle weakness
B. Mild increase in urine output
C. Slight decrease in blood pressure
D. Occasional dizziness after position change
Q430. When implementing infection control for a patient with C. difficile, which measure is essential?
A. Wash hands with soap and water after care
B. Use alcohol-based sanitizer exclusively
C. Dispose linens in regular laundry bins
D. Share equipment among infected patients
Q431. When implementing care for a patient with anemia, which dietary advice supports treatment?
A. Skip supplements when feeling well
B. Avoid meat and green vegetables
C. Increase caffeine intake to reduce fatigue
D. Eat foods rich in iron and vitamin C
Q432. When implementing care for a patient after myocardial infarction, which nursing action is a priority?
A. Monitor for chest pain and administer oxygen
B. Encourage immediate physical activity
C. Provide a high-sodium, high-fat diet
D. Withhold all prescribed medications
Q433. When implementing care for a patient with hypoglycemia, which intervention should the nurse perform first?

A. Give 15 g of fast-acting carbohydrate
B. Notify the healthcare provider immediately
C. Administer long-acting insulin
D. Offer a high-protein meal

Q434. When implementing care for a patient receiving enteral nutrition, which observation requires intervention?
A. Gastric residual of 300 mL
B. Soft, non-distended abdomen
C. Normal bowel sounds present
D. Patient positioned with head elevated

Q435. When implementing care for a patient with postoperative wound drainage, which nursing action is appropriate?
A. Keep the drainage system above incision level
B. Discard output without assessing
C. Disconnect tubing for easier ambulation
D. Measure and document drainage amount and color

Q436. When implementing fall prevention in a confused patient, which strategy is best?
A. Use a bed alarm and frequent safety checks
B. Restrain the patient to prevent movement
C. Keep lights off to encourage sleep
D. Place the call light out of reach

Q437. When implementing care for a patient with peripheral arterial disease, which intervention promotes tissue perfusion?
A. Keep legs dependent when sitting
B. Apply tight compression bandages
C. Elevate legs above heart level
D. Use cold compresses for comfort

Q438. When implementing care for a patient with renal failure, which dietary restriction is appropriate?
A. Limit protein, sodium, and potassium intake
B. Encourage high-protein foods to rebuild muscle
C. Increase dairy and fruit juices
D. Add salt substitutes freely

Q439. When implementing care for a patient with chronic liver disease, which nursing action prevents complications?
A. Avoid measuring abdominal girth daily
B. Encourage alcohol in moderation
C. Provide high-fat foods to increase calories
D. Monitor for signs of bleeding and bruising

Q440. When implementing care for a patient with COPD receiving oxygen therapy, which finding requires intervention?
A. Respiratory rate decreases to 8 breaths/min
B. O_2 saturation 90% on prescribed flow
C. Productive cough of clear sputum
D. Mild dyspnea with exertion

Q441. When implementing teaching for a patient with osteoporosis, which instruction is appropriate?
A. Engage in regular weight-bearing exercise
B. Avoid calcium supplements to prevent stones

C. Limit sunlight exposure
D. Restrict protein intake

Q442. When implementing infection control for a patient with varicella (chickenpox), which precautions are required?
A. Airborne and contact precautions
B. Droplet precautions only
C. Standard precautions only
D. Reverse isolation precautions

Q443. When implementing postoperative care for a patient after appendectomy, which finding requires immediate reporting?
A. Small amount of serosanguinous drainage
B. Mild incisional tenderness
C. Passage of flatus on day two
D. Increasing abdominal pain and rigidity

Q444. When implementing care for a patient with diabetic foot ulcers, which intervention supports healing?
A. Keep ulcers clean and apply prescribed dressings
B. Soak feet in hot water daily
C. Walk barefoot to air out the wounds
D. Apply pressure dressings to stop drainage

Q445. When implementing care for a patient receiving anticoagulant therapy, which finding requires urgent attention?
A. Presence of black, tarry stools
B. Occasional bruising on arms
C. Slight gum bleeding when brushing
D. Mild fatigue after exertion

Q446. When implementing care for a patient after hip replacement, which activity should be avoided?
A. Crossing legs while sitting
B. Using an abduction pillow while in bed
C. Sitting on a raised toilet seat
D. Maintaining neutral leg alignment

Q447. When implementing care for a patient after thyroid surgery, which finding requires immediate intervention?
A. Slight incisional swelling
B. Mild sore throat
C. Small amount of serosanguinous drainage
D. Hoarseness and difficulty breathing

Q448. When implementing care for a patient with chronic renal failure, which dietary modification is appropriate?
A. Limit protein and potassium intake
B. Encourage high-protein meals
C. Increase sodium intake
D. Provide unrestricted dairy products

Q449. When implementing postoperative care for a patient after cataract extraction, which instruction should the nurse reinforce?
A. Avoid bending or lifting heavy objects
B. Rub the affected eye gently to relieve itching
C. Sleep on the operated side for comfort

D. Remove eye shield the same day

Q450. When implementing care for a patient with pneumonia, which position promotes optimal oxygenation?

A. Semi-Fowler's position
B. Supine position
C. Trendelenburg position
D. High-Fowler's with head flexed forward

Q451. When implementing care for a patient receiving IV therapy, which measure prevents phlebitis?

A. Flush with dextrose between infusions
B. Use the same site until occlusion occurs
C. Secure tubing tightly with adhesive tape
D. Rotate IV sites every 72–96 hours

Q452. When implementing care for a patient with COPD, which intervention reduces dyspnea during activity?

A. Teach pursed-lip breathing technique
B. Encourage breath-holding during exertion
C. Increase supplemental oxygen to maximum
D. Instruct on shallow rapid breathing

Q453. When implementing postoperative care for a patient after bowel resection, which finding requires immediate attention?

A. Absent bowel sounds and rigid abdomen
B. Mild distention on day two
C. Small amount of serosanguinous drainage
D. Gradual appetite return

Q454. When implementing care for a patient receiving chemotherapy, which nursing action minimizes infection risk?

A. Encourage meticulous hand hygiene
B. Provide fresh fruits daily for nutrition
C. Administer live vaccines for immunity
D. Limit oral care to once daily

Q455. When implementing care for a patient after abdominal hysterectomy, which intervention promotes venous return?

A. Keep legs elevated on pillows constantly
B. Maintain bedrest until discharge
C. Restrict fluids for 24 hours
D. Encourage early ambulation and leg exercises

Q456. When implementing care for a patient with anemia, which assessment indicates treatment effectiveness?

A. Increased energy and improved pallor
B. Decreased appetite and mild dizziness
C. Persistent fatigue and low pulse rate
D. Pale conjunctiva and tachycardia

Q457. When implementing care for a patient receiving opioid analgesics, which safety measure is essential?

A. Monitor respiratory rate and sedation level
B. Encourage driving after each dose
C. Administer medication without assessing pain
D. Omit documentation of side effects

Q458. When implementing discharge teaching for a diabetic patient, which instruction prevents hypoglycemia?
A. Eat regular meals and carry a quick glucose source
B. Skip meals if blood sugar is high
C. Exercise vigorously without snacks
D. Double insulin dose if symptoms occur
Q459. When implementing care for a patient with fluid overload, which finding signals improvement?
A. Rapid heart rate and orthopnea
B. Weight gain and jugular distention
C. Crackles and increased dyspnea
D. Decreased peripheral edema and clearer breath sounds
Q460. When implementing teaching for a patient on anticoagulation therapy, which statement reflects understanding?
A. "I'll use an electric razor for shaving."
B. "I'll take double doses if I miss one."
C. "I can play contact sports carefully."
D. "I'll stop the drug before every trip."
Q461. When implementing care for a patient with congestive heart failure, which intervention supports fluid management?
A. Weigh the patient daily at the same time
B. Increase sodium intake for balance
C. Limit activity to conserve energy entirely
D. Restrict medication to alternate days
Q462. When implementing care for a patient receiving blood transfusion, which nursing action ensures safety?
A. Verify blood type and patient ID with another nurse
B. Use dextrose solution to prime the IV line
C. Begin infusion without crossmatch
D. Leave patient unattended during first 15 minutes
Q463. When implementing care for a patient after stroke, which intervention promotes independence?
A. Avoid mobility exercises early
B. Provide total care to prevent fatigue
C. Limit participation in daily activities
D. Encourage use of the unaffected hand for self-care
Q464. When implementing care for a patient with hypertension, which teaching should the nurse emphasize?
A. Limit sodium and alcohol intake
B. Discontinue medication when blood pressure improves
C. Avoid moderate physical activity
D. Increase processed food consumption
Q465. When implementing care for a patient with chronic pain, which nursing action best supports coping?
A. Encourage relaxation and distraction techniques
B. Focus discussion only on medication effects
C. Discourage expression of discomfort
D. Limit emotional support during assessments

Q466. When implementing postoperative teaching for a patient after laminectomy, which instruction is correct?
A. Avoid twisting or bending at the waist
B. Sit upright for long periods
C. Sleep on the stomach for comfort
D. Lift light objects immediately after surgery
Q467. When implementing care for a patient receiving blood transfusion, which finding requires immediate action?
A. Feeling tired post-transfusion
B. Mild headache near completion
C. Slight warmth at IV site
D. Back pain and chills during infusion
Q468. When implementing postoperative care for a patient after hysterectomy, which intervention promotes bowel function?
A. Encourage early ambulation and fluid intake
B. Restrict oral fluids for 48 hours
C. Provide narcotics liberally for pain
D. Maintain bedrest until bowel sounds return
Q469. When implementing care for a patient on chemotherapy, which precaution reduces bleeding risk?
A. Use a soft toothbrush and avoid invasive procedures
B. Perform deep tissue massage to prevent clots
C. Use rectal thermometers for accuracy
D. Administer aspirin for pain relief
Q470. When implementing teaching for a patient with diabetes, which foot care instruction is essential?
A. Check feet daily for cuts or blisters
B. Use heating pads to keep feet warm
C. Trim toenails deeply to prevent ingrown nails
D. Walk barefoot to improve circulation
Q471. When implementing care for a patient with hypovolemia, which finding shows effective fluid replacement?
A. Decreased capillary refill
B. Jugular vein distention
C. Crackles in the lungs
D. Improved blood pressure and urine output
Q472. When implementing infection control for a patient with influenza, which precautions are required?
A. Droplet precautions
B. Contact precautions only
C. Airborne isolation
D. Reverse isolation
Q473. When implementing care for a patient with urinary retention, which intervention aids bladder emptying?
A. Run warm water or pour water over the perineum
B. Maintain strict fluid restriction
C. Encourage holding urine until urgency returns
D. Avoid any bladder stimulation techniques

Q474. When implementing care for a patient on digoxin therapy, which assessment ensures safety?
A. Check apical pulse before administration
B. Assess radial pulse only once daily
C. Administer even if pulse is irregular
D. Skip documentation after each dose
Q475. When implementing care for a patient with COPD, which instruction optimizes oxygen therapy?
A. Use humidifier only when coughing
B. Increase flow when short of breath
C. Remove nasal cannula while sleeping
D. Use prescribed flow rate only
Q476. When implementing postoperative care for a patient after cataract surgery, which activity is contraindicated?
A. Bending forward to pick up items
B. Using stool softeners for constipation
C. Wearing protective eyewear outdoors
D. Sleeping on the nonoperative side
Q477. When implementing care for a patient with ascites, which nursing action helps reduce fluid accumulation?
A. Restrict sodium intake
B. Encourage high-salt foods
C. Promote large fluid intake
D. Limit daily weight measurements
Q478. When implementing care for a patient with an NG tube for suction, which observation indicates a complication?
A. Absence of gastric drainage and distention
B. Greenish drainage with audible suction
C. Flat abdomen with no pain
D. Air bubbles in collection tubing
Q479. When implementing care for a patient after hip surgery, which safety measure prevents dislocation?
A. Sit on low chairs or stools
B. Cross legs while turning in bed
C. Bend hip beyond 90 degrees
D. Maintain legs in abduction using pillows
Q480. When implementing care for a patient with diabetes insipidus, which nursing action is most important?
A. Monitor urine output and specific gravity closely
B. Restrict fluids to prevent overload
C. Encourage high-sodium diet
D. Administer insulin before meals
Q481. When implementing discharge teaching for a patient with heart failure, which statement indicates understanding?
A. "I'll weigh myself every morning at the same time."
B. "I'll take an extra diuretic dose if I gain weight."
C. "I'll limit rest to strengthen my heart."
D. "I'll skip medication when swelling decreases."
Q482. When implementing care for a patient with pressure injuries, which intervention promotes healing?

A. Reposition every two hours
B. Massage reddened skin to increase blood flow
C. Keep the area dry and uncovered
D. Avoid nutritional supplementation

Q483. When implementing infection control for a patient with tuberculosis, which precaution is necessary?

A. No isolation needed after antibiotic initiation
B. Use surgical mask and open window
C. Apply contact precautions only
D. Use N95 respirator and negative-pressure room

Q484. When implementing care for a patient on anticoagulation therapy, which instruction ensures safety?

A. Avoid foods high in vitamin K
B. Take medication at different times daily
C. Stop medication during menses
D. Ignore signs of bleeding

Q485. When implementing postoperative care after colon surgery, which assessment requires urgent attention?

A. Absent bowel sounds and increasing pain
B. Serosanguinous drainage from incision
C. Mild abdominal distention
D. Gradual appetite improvement

Q486. When implementing teaching for a patient prescribed diuretics, which instruction supports safe self-care?

A. Change positions slowly to prevent dizziness
B. Increase sodium intake to replace losses
C. Skip doses if feeling well
D. Avoid daily weight monitoring

Q487. When implementing care for a patient with heart failure on furosemide, which assessment requires priority?

A. Skin turgor on hands
B. Pupil reaction to light
C. Bowel movement frequency
D. Serum potassium level

Q488. When implementing teaching for a patient after mastectomy, which instruction is correct?

A. Perform gentle arm exercises on the affected side
B. Keep the affected arm immobile at all times
C. Avoid wearing prescribed compression garments
D. Measure arm circumference only once yearly

Q489. When implementing care for a patient with diabetic ketoacidosis, which intervention is the initial priority?

A. Administer IV fluids as prescribed
B. Start long-acting insulin immediately
C. Provide oral fluids for hydration
D. Restrict glucose monitoring

Q490. When implementing care for a patient receiving a transfusion, which action ensures safety during the first 15 minutes?

A. Remain with the patient and monitor for reactions

B. Increase infusion rate to full speed
C. Administer medication through the same line
D. Leave the patient unattended briefly

Q491. When implementing postoperative teaching for a patient after spinal fusion, which activity should be avoided?

A. Wearing a prescribed back brace
B. Using a firm mattress for support
C. Logrolling when repositioning
D. Bending or twisting the spine

Q492. When implementing care for a patient with dehydration, which urine characteristic indicates improvement?

A. Pale yellow color and specific gravity near 1.015
B. Dark amber color and high specific gravity
C. Cloudy urine with odor
D. No change in volume after fluid replacement

Q493. When implementing teaching for a patient on corticosteroid therapy, which precaution should the nurse emphasize?

A. Avoid abrupt discontinuation of medication
B. Restrict dietary protein
C. Take medication on an empty stomach
D. Double dose if stress increases

Q494. When implementing care for a patient with a tracheostomy, which assessment finding requires immediate action?

A. Absence of airflow and difficulty breathing
B. Small amount of clear mucus at site
C. Slight hoarseness after suctioning
D. Moist skin around stoma

Q495. When implementing care for a patient after abdominal surgery, which intervention prevents pulmonary complications?

A. Delay ambulation until day three
B. Maintain supine position for rest
C. Limit coughing to reduce pain
D. Encourage incentive spirometry every hour

Q496. When implementing infection control for a patient with MRSA, which precaution is essential?

A. Use contact precautions and dedicated equipment
B. Share thermometers between patients
C. Remove gloves before leaving the room only
D. Use airborne isolation exclusively

Q497. When implementing care for a patient on enteral feedings, which action prevents aspiration?

A. Elevate head of bed 30–45 degrees
B. Flush tubing once daily only
C. Administer feeding with patient supine
D. Ignore residual volume checks

Q498. When implementing care for a patient with hyperkalemia, which medication supports correction?

A. Administer insulin with glucose as prescribed
B. Give potassium supplements
C. Use potassium-sparing diuretics

D. Restrict IV fluids

Q499. When implementing care for a patient with pneumonia, which outcome indicates improvement?

A. Labored breathing and cyanosis

B. Persistent cough with thick sputum

C. Decreased temperature and clear breath sounds

D. Productive cough with blood-streaked sputum

Q500. When implementing postoperative care after hip replacement, which activity should the patient avoid?

A. Crossing legs or bending beyond 90 degrees

B. Using a high toilet seat

C. Keeping legs in slight abduction

D. Sitting with knees apart

Answer key and Explanation (401-500)

Q401. Answer: A

Explanation: Distention with rigidity and pain suggests internal bleeding or peritonitis, requiring emergency evaluation. Mild tenderness and delayed bowel sounds are expected. Early recognition of abdominal complications prevents sepsis and maintains hemodynamic stability.

Q402. Answer: A

Explanation: Isotonic saline replaces extracellular volume rapidly, restoring perfusion. Dextrose solutions do not correct sodium loss, and LR may follow stabilization. Immediate isotonic replacement treats hypovolemia safely and supports circulatory function.

Q403. Answer: A

Explanation: Gradual arm exercises prevent stiffness and promote lymphatic drainage. Restriction delays mobility and healing. Tight bandages impair circulation. Controlled activity restores function and prevents lymphedema complications after breast surgery.

Q404. Answer: D

Explanation: Hand hygiene remains the most effective infection control measure. Gloves supplement but never replace it. Reusing PPE or skipping washing spreads pathogens. Clean hands before and after care protect both patients and staff universally.

Q405. Answer: A

Explanation: Validating acknowledges pain as real, fostering trust and open communication. Ignoring subjective reports or minimizing complaints damages rapport. Patient-centered empathy and education form the foundation of effective chronic pain management and adherence.

Q406. Answer: A

Explanation: Coughing and deep breathing promote secretion mobilization and lung expansion. Fluid restriction and sedation hinder clearance, while movement aids ventilation. Airway management focuses on secretion control and oxygen optimization for respiratory recovery.

Q407. Answer: A

Explanation: Keeping the patient NPO minimizes pancreatic stimulation and enzyme release, reducing inflammation. Early oral intake worsens pain, and high-fat foods increase enzyme secretion. IV fluids prevent hypovolemia, while heat may aggravate discomfort. Resting the pancreas is essential for recovery.

Q408. Answer: D

Explanation: Bananas and potatoes are rich in potassium and restore normal serum levels. Rice, toast, and low-potassium foods provide little correction. Proper dietary teaching complements medication therapy in treating hypokalemia and maintaining electrolyte balance.

Q409. Answer: A

Explanation: Emptying the pouch when one-third full prevents leakage and discomfort. Alcohol irritates the skin, and fluid intake must increase to prevent dehydration. Pouches are replaced regularly for hygiene. Proper stoma care supports comfort and skin integrity.

Q410. Answer: A

Explanation: Logrolling maintains spinal alignment and prevents stress on the surgical site. Unsupported sitting and twisting strain the spine, risking injury or hardware displacement. Controlled movements preserve integrity, reduce pain, and promote safe healing after spinal procedures.

Q411. Answer: D

Explanation: Hypocalcemia increases neuromuscular excitability, predisposing to seizures. Safety precautions are essential. Phosphorus worsens calcium deficit, and loop diuretics promote calcium loss. Adequate calcium intake and supplementation restore balance and prevent complications such as tetany.

Q412. Answer: A

Explanation: Frequent glucose monitoring detects hyperglycemia, a common TPN effect. Abrupt discontinuation causes rebound hypoglycemia. TPN solutions are replaced every 24 hours to reduce infection risk. Dedicated central line care maintains sterility and infusion consistency.

Q413. Answer: A

Explanation: Gradual tapering prevents adrenal insufficiency from abrupt withdrawal. Steroids should be taken with food to prevent gastric irritation. Mood changes are significant side effects requiring evaluation. Gradual discontinuation ensures endocrine stability and safe withdrawal.

Q414. Answer: A

Explanation: Sterile suctioning prevents introduction of pathogens into the airway. Tap water and self-tie changes risk contamination and displacement. Humidified air maintains secretion mobility. Strict asepsis and teamwork reduce respiratory infection risk in tracheostomy care.

Q415. Answer: D

Explanation: Rash and respiratory distress suggest anaphylaxis, requiring immediate discontinuation and emergency response. Mild nausea or warmth are common, non-life-threatening reactions. Early detection of hypersensitivity ensures prompt treatment and prevention of systemic complications.

Q416. Answer: A

Explanation: Compression devices enhance venous return, preventing clot formation. Bedrest increases DVT risk, and fluid restriction hinders circulation. Early, safe leg exercises complement prevention efforts. Combining mobility with compression promotes vascular health postoperatively.

Q417. Answer: A

Explanation: Gravity drainage requires the system to remain below chest level. Clamping or stripping can create high pressure, risking lung injury. The collection chamber is not emptied but replaced when full. Proper setup maintains safe pleural drainage.

Q418. Answer: A

Explanation: Monitoring sedation and respiratory rate detects early signs of depression. Overdosing or sedative combination increases risk. Naloxone is the antidote for significant respiratory compromise, not cardiac events. Vigilant assessment ensures opioid safety and comfort balance.

Q419. Answer: C

Explanation: Sodium restriction and regular activity lower blood pressure effectively. Inconsistent medication use or processed foods worsen hypertension. Potassium moderation depends on medication type. Lifestyle adherence strengthens pharmacologic therapy outcomes and cardiovascular health.

Q420. Answer: A

Explanation: Elevating the head reduces aspiration risk and improves ventilation. Disabling alarms or routine saline use compromises airway protection. Minimal restraints support safety only if needed. Proper positioning ensures effective oxygenation and reduces ventilator-associated pneumonia risk.

Q421. Answer: A

Explanation: Chest pain post-CABG may indicate graft occlusion or ischemia requiring urgent evaluation. Heavy lifting strains the sternum, and stopping medications risks reinfarction. Persistent fever signals infection, not normal recovery. Education promotes vigilance and safe healing.

Q422. Answer: A

Explanation: Placement verification prevents aspiration and ensures proper delivery. Mixing drugs with feedings alters absorption, and infrequent flushing clogs tubing. Supine positioning heightens aspiration risk. Verification and head elevation maintain safety during enteral therapy.

Q423. Answer: D

Explanation: Oral or hypotonic fluid intake restores balance and reduces serum sodium levels. Hypertonic solutions worsen hypernatremia. Dietary sodium restriction supports therapy. Gradual correction prevents cerebral edema and neurological complications in sodium imbalance management.

Q424. Answer: A

Explanation: Securing the catheter prevents urethral traction and injury. Elevating or disconnecting tubing introduces infection risk. Routine flushing is unnecessary unless ordered. Proper stabilization and aseptic care ensure safe urinary drainage and comfort.

Q425. Answer: A

Explanation: Elevation facilitates venous outflow and reduces ICP. Coughing and flexion elevate pressure, and hypotonic fluids worsen cerebral edema. Head elevation with neutral alignment optimizes cerebral perfusion and protects brain tissue.

Q426. Answer: A

Explanation: Early ambulation and hydration stimulate peristalsis and prevent ileus. Prolonged fasting delays recovery, and immobility promotes complications. Spirometry supports oxygenation, not bowel function. Gradual mobility aids gastrointestinal motility restoration safely.

Q427. Answer: C

Explanation: Ambulation stimulates bile movement and prevents postoperative ileus. Prolonged bedrest increases risk for respiratory and circulatory complications. Adequate fluids and gradual diet progression support recovery. Early mobilization accelerates healing and improves gastrointestinal function.

Q428. Answer: A

Explanation: Deep breathing and coughing expand alveoli and remove mucus, improving oxygenation. Supine positioning and fluid restriction hinder secretion mobilization. Hydration and upright posture optimize lung ventilation and promote effective airway clearance.

Q429. Answer: A

Explanation: Irregular rhythm and weakness suggest hypokalemia, a serious side effect of diuretics. Mild hypotension and dizziness are expected but monitored. Electrolyte imbalance may cause arrhythmias, requiring prompt correction to ensure cardiac safety during diuretic therapy.

Q430. Answer: A

Explanation: C. difficile spores resist alcohol; handwashing physically removes them. Dedicated equipment and special linen handling prevent spread. Sanitizers alone are ineffective. Strict contact precautions maintain safety and limit environmental contamination.

Q431. Answer: D

Explanation: Iron and vitamin C improve hemoglobin synthesis and absorption. Avoiding nutrient-rich foods worsens anemia, and caffeine inhibits absorption. Consistent dietary compliance ensures red blood cell restoration and energy improvement during treatment.

Q432. Answer: A

Explanation: Oxygen and pain control reduce myocardial workload and prevent further ischemia. Early exertion or poor diet increases stress on the heart. Adherence to prescribed therapy and monitoring support cardiac recovery and stability post-MI.

Q433. Answer: A

Explanation: Rapid glucose administration restores levels and relieves symptoms quickly. Protein or insulin worsens hypoglycemia. Provider notification follows if the patient fails to respond. Early carbohydrate treatment prevents neurological injury and hypoglycemic shock.

Q434. Answer: A

Explanation: High residual volume indicates delayed gastric emptying, increasing aspiration risk. Non-distended abdomen and normal sounds are expected. Proper positioning promotes digestion. Regular residual checks and feeding adjustment prevent regurgitation and aspiration pneumonia.

Q435. Answer: D

Explanation: Monitoring drainage provides data on healing and potential complications. Disconnection introduces infection, and elevation prevents gravity flow. Accurate documentation guides evaluation of wound healing and early detection of abnormal bleeding or infection.

Q436. Answer: A

Explanation: Bed alarms and checks promote supervision while maintaining dignity. Restraints and poor lighting increase confusion and fall risk. Accessible call lights encourage patient engagement in safety. Proactive observation ensures effective prevention without restricting mobility.

Q437. Answer: A

Explanation: Dependent leg positioning enhances arterial flow to extremities. Elevation impairs perfusion, and compression worsens ischemia. Heat application, not cold, relieves pain and encourages circulation. Proper positioning improves comfort and tissue oxygenation.

Q438. Answer: A

Explanation: Protein, sodium, and potassium restriction prevent waste buildup and electrolyte imbalance. Excess protein strains kidneys, and salt substitutes often contain potassium. Controlled diet management supports renal function and reduces metabolic complications.

Q439. Answer: D

Explanation: Liver dysfunction impairs clotting; monitoring bleeding identifies complications early. Alcohol worsens hepatic damage, and fatty foods increase stress on digestion. Measuring abdominal girth detects ascites progression. Vigilant assessment supports stability and early intervention.

Q440. Answer: A

Explanation: Depressed respirations indicate oxygen-induced hypoventilation, a dangerous side effect in COPD. Saturations near 90% are acceptable. Mild dyspnea is expected. Oxygen must be titrated carefully to maintain hypoxic drive while supporting adequate ventilation.

Q441. Answer: A

Explanation: Weight-bearing activity strengthens bone density and reduces fracture risk. Adequate calcium and vitamin D are essential. Sunlight promotes vitamin D synthesis, not harm. Balanced nutrition and exercise prevent progression of osteoporosis effectively.

Q442. Answer: A

Explanation: Varicella spreads through airborne droplets and direct contact. Dual precautions prevent hospital transmission. Standard measures alone are insufficient, and reverse isolation protects immunocompromised, not infectious patients. Isolation continues until lesions crust over completely.

Q443. Answer: D

Explanation: Worsening pain and rigidity signal possible peritonitis or abscess formation. Mild tenderness and minor drainage are normal postoperative findings. Prompt evaluation prevents sepsis and promotes timely surgical intervention if complications arise.

Q444. Answer: A

Explanation: Clean dressings prevent infection and support tissue repair. Hot water and pressure cause burns or impaired circulation. Protective footwear and regular inspection reduce injury risk. Consistent care promotes wound healing and prevents amputation.

Q445. Answer: A

Explanation: Black stools indicate gastrointestinal bleeding, a serious anticoagulation complication. Mild bruising or gum bleeding may occur but should still be monitored. Early detection of internal bleeding prevents hemorrhagic shock and ensures patient safety.

Q446. Answer: A

Explanation: Crossing legs causes hip dislocation by promoting internal rotation. Abduction pillows, alignment, and raised seating maintain joint safety. Patient education on posture and movement restrictions prevents prosthesis displacement and ensures stable recovery.

Q447. Answer: D

Explanation: Hoarseness and breathing difficulty suggest airway obstruction from hematoma or laryngeal nerve injury. Minor soreness and drainage are expected postoperative findings. Prompt airway assessment and emergency equipment readiness prevent respiratory compromise after thyroidectomy.

Q448. Answer: A

Explanation: Restricted protein and potassium intake minimize uremic toxin buildup and prevent hyperkalemia. Excess sodium and dairy worsen fluid and electrolyte imbalance. Tailored nutrition supports renal function preservation and stabilizes metabolic homeostasis in chronic disease.

Q449. Answer: A

Explanation: Avoiding bending or lifting prevents intraocular pressure increase and protects surgical integrity. Rubbing or sleeping on the operated side risks trauma. The protective shield remains until advised. Careful positioning ensures proper healing and vision preservation.

Q450. Answer: A

Explanation: Semi-Fowler's improves lung expansion and ventilation-perfusion balance. Supine and Trendelenburg hinder diaphragmatic movement, while excessive flexion strains the airway. Upright positioning supports oxygen exchange and patient comfort in respiratory management.

Q451. Answer: D

Explanation: Regular site rotation minimizes vein irritation and infection. Continuous use damages vessel walls, and tight taping impedes circulation. Saline flushing maintains patency safely. Preventive rotation and monitoring preserve venous integrity during therapy.

Q452. Answer: A

Explanation: Pursed-lip breathing prolongs exhalation, preventing air trapping and reducing dyspnea. Rapid or breath-holding patterns worsen gas exchange. Oxygen titration follows prescription. Controlled breathing techniques improve endurance and respiratory efficiency in COPD management.

Q453. Answer: A

Explanation: Rigidity and absent bowel sounds indicate possible peritonitis or obstruction, a surgical emergency. Mild distention and drainage are typical early findings. Timely recognition prevents sepsis and ensures swift medical intervention for abdominal complications.

Q454. Answer: A

Explanation: Hand hygiene is critical for immunocompromised patients to prevent infection. Fresh produce and live vaccines expose pathogens. Frequent gentle oral care prevents mucosal breakdown. Infection control protects patient safety during cytotoxic therapy.

Q455. Answer: D

Explanation: Early movement and leg exercises prevent venous stasis and thrombosis. Prolonged bedrest delays circulation, and continuous elevation may reduce comfort. Adequate fluids and ambulation enhance recovery and lower postoperative DVT risk.

Q456. Answer: A

Explanation: Improved pallor and energy reflect rising hemoglobin levels and oxygen delivery. Fatigue and pallor suggest ongoing anemia. Monitoring clinical improvement validates therapeutic response and helps guide nutritional or pharmacologic interventions.

Q457. Answer: A

Explanation: Continuous respiratory and sedation assessment ensures early detection of overdose or depression. Driving impairs safety, and assessment guides proper dosing. Documentation supports monitoring and communication among the healthcare team for patient safety.

Q458. Answer: A

Explanation: Consistent meals and emergency glucose prevent dangerous drops. Skipping meals or extra insulin causes severe hypoglycemia. Patient education on symptoms and timing promotes safe glucose regulation and self-care confidence.

Q459. Answer: D

Explanation: Reduced edema and clear lungs show successful diuretic therapy and fluid balance. Weight gain and crackles indicate persistent overload. Continuous monitoring of respiratory and circulatory responses confirms treatment progress and stability.

Q460. Answer: A

Explanation: Electric razors minimize bleeding risk. Doubling doses or stopping abruptly causes instability. Contact sports are contraindicated. Reinforcing lifestyle adjustments and adherence prevents hemorrhage and thrombotic events in anticoagulated patients.

Q461. Answer: A

Explanation: Daily weights track subtle fluid changes, guiding treatment. Sodium restriction and medication consistency prevent exacerbation. Complete inactivity reduces circulation. Routine monitoring provides early detection of retention and aids management adjustments.

Q462. Answer: A

Explanation: Two-nurse verification prevents transfusion mismatch. Dextrose hemolyzes red cells, and lack of crossmatch risks reaction. Close observation early detects adverse events quickly, ensuring patient safety and transfusion accuracy.

Q463. Answer: D

Explanation: Using the unaffected side supports adaptation and confidence in recovery. Total dependence hinders rehabilitation, and immobility increases complications. Gradual, guided practice fosters functional restoration and psychosocial well-being.

Q464. Answer: A

Explanation: Sodium and alcohol restriction maintain vascular tone and blood pressure control. Stopping medication or consuming processed foods causes rebound hypertension. Consistent lifestyle adherence complements drug therapy for optimal outcomes.

Q465. Answer: A

Explanation: Relaxation and distraction empower patients and reduce pain perception. Open communication enhances trust. Limiting emotional support or discussion isolates patients. Integrating nonpharmacologic methods strengthens holistic pain control and well-being.

Q466. Answer: A

Explanation: Twisting stresses the spine and surgical repair site. Prolonged sitting and early lifting delay healing. Logrolling and posture support alignment, preventing reinjury and promoting spinal stabilization during recovery.

Q467. Answer: D

Explanation: Chills and back pain indicate a hemolytic reaction, requiring immediate transfusion stop and emergency response. Mild headache and fatigue can occur normally. Early recognition and prompt action prevent shock, renal failure, and severe systemic complications.

Q468. Answer: A

Explanation: Ambulation and hydration stimulate peristalsis and prevent ileus. Prolonged fasting and immobility slow recovery. Excess opioids cause constipation. Early movement safely restores gastrointestinal function and supports recovery following abdominal surgery.

Q469. Answer: A

Explanation: Thrombocytopenia increases bleeding risk; soft hygiene and avoiding trauma prevent hemorrhage. Rectal procedures and aspirin exacerbate bleeding. Gentle care and medication review ensure safety for immunosuppressed oncology patients during active chemotherapy.

Q470. Answer: A

Explanation: Daily inspection detects early injury, preventing ulcers and infection. Heating pads and barefoot walking increase burn and trauma risk. Gentle trimming and protective footwear maintain safety and prevent diabetic foot complications.

Q471. Answer: D

Explanation: Stable vitals and adequate urine indicate restored volume. Distention and crackles suggest overload, while poor refill implies persistent deficit. Close assessment confirms balanced rehydration and effective circulatory function restoration.

Q472. Answer: A

Explanation: Influenza spreads via respiratory droplets; masks and distance prevent transmission. Airborne and contact precautions are excessive. Reverse isolation protects immunocompromised individuals, not infected ones. Adherence to droplet protocol ensures infection containment.

Q473. Answer: A

Explanation: Warm water promotes relaxation of the urinary sphincter, facilitating voiding. Fluid restriction and delayed urination worsen retention. Noninvasive stimulation is first-line management before catheterization, supporting safe and effective bladder emptying.

Q474. Answer: A

Explanation: Apical pulse monitoring detects bradycardia or irregular rhythm, preventing toxicity. Skipping assessments or documentation compromises safety. Dose should be withheld for low pulse rate. Continuous monitoring supports therapeutic and safe cardiac management.

Q475. Answer: D

Explanation: Oxygen flow must remain at the ordered rate to prevent hypoventilation. Overuse suppresses respiratory drive. Consistent usage and humidification prevent dryness and maintain safe oxygenation. Adherence ensures stability and respiratory efficiency.

Q476. Answer: A

Explanation: Bending increases intraocular pressure, risking surgical disruption. Stool softeners and protective gear promote healing. Sleeping on the opposite side avoids pressure. Safe positioning and activity modification preserve vision recovery post-surgery.

Q477. Answer: A

Explanation: Sodium restriction reduces fluid retention and ascitic buildup. High salt and excess fluids worsen imbalance. Daily weights track fluid status. Nutritional control and diuretics together manage cirrhotic fluid overload effectively.

Q478. Answer: A

Explanation: Lack of output with distention suggests obstruction or tube displacement. Green drainage indicates normal bile suction. Timely evaluation and repositioning prevent perforation, aspiration, and abdominal pressure complications during gastric decompression.

Q479. Answer: D

Explanation: Abduction alignment prevents hip dislocation postoperatively. Crossing legs or excessive flexion strains the joint. Raised seating ensures safety. Maintaining proper positioning protects the surgical repair and supports stable mobility recovery.

Q480. Answer: A

Explanation: Excessive dilute urine output reflects ADH deficiency; monitoring evaluates therapy effectiveness. Restricting fluids risks dehydration, and insulin is unrelated. Tracking output and lab values ensures prompt correction and electrolyte stability.

Q481. Answer: A

Explanation: Daily weights detect early fluid retention. Extra dosing or medication omission causes instability. Balance between rest and activity maintains strength. Self-monitoring and adherence prevent hospital readmission and support long-term heart failure management.

Q482. Answer: A

Explanation: Repositioning prevents tissue ischemia and further breakdown. Massaging inflamed areas causes damage. Moist, protected environments and adequate nutrition promote repair. Frequent repositioning remains the cornerstone of pressure injury management.

Q483. Answer: D

Explanation: TB requires airborne precautions with a respirator and negative pressure to prevent spread. Surgical masks are inadequate. Isolation remains until sputum tests confirm noninfectious status. Proper protocols protect healthcare workers and others.

Q484. Answer: A

Explanation: Vitamin K interferes with anticoagulant effects; dietary consistency is vital. Irregular timing and discontinuation cause fluctuation. Reporting bleeding ensures prompt intervention. Patient education reduces complications and maintains therapeutic stability.

Q485. Answer: A

Explanation: Pain with silent bowel sounds indicates ileus or obstruction, needing immediate evaluation. Minor drainage and mild distention are expected initially. Continuous assessment allows early detection of life-threatening abdominal complications.

Q486. Answer: A

Explanation: Slow movement prevents postural hypotension, a common diuretic effect. Skipping doses or adding sodium disrupts fluid balance. Regular weight checks detect fluid changes. Safety education ensures adherence and prevents dehydration or electrolyte imbalance.

Q487. Answer: D

Explanation: Furosemide can cause hypokalemia, leading to arrhythmias. Monitoring potassium ensures electrolyte stability. Pupil response and bowel frequency are unrelated to diuretic therapy. Regular laboratory evaluation maintains cardiac rhythm safety and medication effectiveness.

Q488. Answer: A

Explanation: Gentle exercises maintain mobility and prevent lymphedema. Immobilization increases stiffness, and compression garments assist fluid drainage. Regular monitoring detects early swelling. Gradual activity supports lymphatic flow and full upper limb recovery.

Q489. Answer: A

Explanation: Rapid IV rehydration corrects hypovolemia and improves perfusion before insulin therapy. Oral fluids are unsafe in altered consciousness. Continuous glucose monitoring guides insulin titration. Fluid resuscitation stabilizes vital function in DKA emergencies.

Q490. Answer: A

Explanation: Reactions typically occur early; close monitoring allows immediate intervention. High infusion rates and drug co-administration risk complications. Continuous presence safeguards against hemolysis, anaphylaxis, or circulatory overload during transfusion initiation.

Q491. Answer: D

Explanation: Bending and twisting stress the fusion site and compromise alignment. Supportive bedding, logrolling, and braces stabilize recovery. Teaching proper movement protects spinal integrity and promotes safe healing postoperatively.

Q492. Answer: A

Explanation: Dilute, light-colored urine shows adequate hydration. Concentrated or odorous urine signals ongoing fluid deficit. Monitoring output verifies effective therapy. Balanced intake and ongoing observation maintain renal perfusion and systemic fluid stability.

Q493. Answer: A

Explanation: Abrupt withdrawal risks adrenal crisis due to suppressed cortisol production. Protein aids tissue repair, and food prevents gastric irritation. Dosing adjustments occur under supervision. Gradual tapering ensures safe endocrine recovery.

Q494. Answer: A

Explanation: Absent airflow indicates obstruction or dislodgement, a life-threatening emergency. Minor secretions and hoarseness are expected. Immediate airway assessment and intervention restore patency. Airway monitoring remains the highest nursing priority in tracheostomy care.

Q495. Answer: D

Explanation: Spirometry promotes lung expansion and secretion clearance, reducing pneumonia risk. Supine positioning and immobility impair ventilation. Pain control supports deep breathing. Early pulmonary exercises enhance oxygenation and recovery efficiency.

Q496. Answer: A

Explanation: MRSA spreads via direct contact; gloves, gowns, and dedicated tools prevent transmission. Shared equipment and improper glove removal increase contamination. Contact isolation maintains safe infection control in healthcare settings.

Q497. Answer: A

Explanation: Elevation facilitates gastric emptying and reduces reflux risk. Supine feeding and poor monitoring increase aspiration danger. Regular flushing maintains patency. Positioning remains the most effective preventive measure for airway safety.

Q498. Answer: A

Explanation: Insulin drives potassium into cells, lowering serum levels. Supplements and sparing diuretics worsen hyperkalemia. IV fluids may aid dilution but are secondary. Prompt medication and monitoring prevent arrhythmias and stabilize cardiac function.

Q499. Answer: C

Explanation: Normalized temperature and clear lungs show infection resolution. Persistent productive or bloody sputum suggests complications. Ongoing assessment ensures therapeutic success and detects potential relapse early during respiratory recovery.

Q500. Answer: A

Explanation: Crossing or deep bending dislocates the prosthesis. Raised seats and abduction positioning maintain alignment. Teaching safe postures prevents joint strain and ensures stable long-term mobility after hip surgery.

Questions (501-600)

Q501. A nurse leader implements evidence-based protocols to reduce catheter-associated infections. Which leadership principle is demonstrated?

A. Transactional management
B. Transformational leadership
C. Laissez-faire supervision
D. Autocratic direction

Q502. A charge nurse encourages staff to reflect on near-miss medication errors during safety huddles. This best represents:

A. Blame-free culture
B. Punitive policy
C. Hierarchical feedback
D. Authoritarian supervision

Q503. A nurse manager assigns an experienced nurse to mentor a new graduate. This action supports which professional standard?

A. Collegiality and collaboration
B. Accountability
C. Autonomy
D. Confidentiality

Q504. A nurse refuses to document care performed by a coworker. This demonstrates:

A. Advocacy
B. Integrity
C. Beneficence
D. Teamwork

Q505. Which action best demonstrates the nurse's role as a patient advocate?

A. Reporting unsafe staffing levels to administration
B. Delegating tasks to unlicensed personnel
C. Completing discharge paperwork promptly
D. Complying silently with physician orders

Q506. A staff nurse reviews updated fall-prevention policies and applies them in care. This behavior reflects:

A. Professional accountability
B. Cultural awareness
C. Empathy
D. Delegation

Q507. A nurse researcher ensures participant confidentiality by coding data instead of using names. Which ethical principle applies?

A. Veracity
B. Justice
C. Fidelity
D. Confidentiality

Q508. A nurse educator schedules competency workshops after identifying skill gaps. This action aligns with:

A. Quality improvement
B. Cost reduction
C. Administrative control
D. Disciplinary action

Q509. A nurse is assigned tasks beyond their scope and respectfully declines. This demonstrates:
A. Professional boundaries
B. Negligence
C. Lack of teamwork
D. Over-delegation
Q510. During an interprofessional meeting, the nurse mediates differing opinions to reach consensus. This illustrates:
A. Collaboration
B. Assertiveness
C. Conflict avoidance
D. Hierarchical leadership
Q511. A nurse manager tracks hand-hygiene compliance monthly to evaluate staff performance. This is an example of:
A. Outcome measurement
B. Peer review
C. Self-assessment
D. Clinical audit
Q512. The nurse's participation in a hospital ethics committee primarily supports which role?
A. Educator
B. Advocate
C. Policy developer
D. Researcher
Q513. A nurse informs a patient about treatment options without bias. This upholds the ethical principle of:
A. Autonomy
B. Nonmaleficence
C. Fidelity
D. Justice
Q514. Which action best demonstrates professional accountability in documentation?
A. Recording care at the end of shift
B. Charting interventions immediately after completion
C. Delegating documentation to assistants
D. Waiting for physician review
Q515. A nurse refuses to share a patient's diagnosis with an unauthorized visitor. This demonstrates:
A. Justice
B. Confidentiality
C. Autonomy
D. Veracity
Q516. A nurse manager encourages staff to report safety concerns without fear of punishment. This promotes:
A. Just culture
B. Bureaucratic control
C. Vertical communication
D. Defensive practice
Q517. A nurse updates personal knowledge by completing annual competency modules. This behavior shows:
A. Lifelong learning
B. Time management

C. Supervision
D. Productivity

Q518. A nurse delegates vital-sign measurement to an unlicensed assistant after confirming competency. This illustrates:

A. Safe delegation
B. Abdication of duty
C. Passive management
D. Task avoidance

Q519. A nurse testifies honestly about clinical actions during a legal case. This demonstrates:

A. Veracity
B. Advocacy
C. Justice
D. Accountability

Q520. A nurse uses hospital data to propose a new discharge-planning protocol. This exemplifies:

A. Intuition
B. Routine procedure
C. Evidence-based practice
D. Administrative compliance

Q521. A nurse participates in writing new infection control policies. This activity represents:

A. Shared governance
B. Delegation
C. Advocacy
D. Case management

Q522. When discussing a patient's prognosis, a nurse provides information using plain, empathetic language. This action demonstrates:

A. Cultural competence
B. Therapeutic communication
C. Passive listening
D. Technical accuracy

Q523. A nurse reports a coworker diverting narcotics. This reflects the ethical principle of:

A. Fidelity
B. Justice
C. Accountability
D. Beneficence

Q524. A nurse leader encourages feedback from team members before changing care procedures. This leadership style is:

A. Democratic
B. Autocratic
C. Transactional
D. Laissez-faire

Q525. A nurse maintains cultural humility when caring for a patient with differing health beliefs by:

A. Exploring the patient's perspective respectfully
B. Correcting misconceptions firmly
C. Avoiding cultural discussion
D. Replacing rituals with evidence-based rules

Q526. A staff nurse leads an in-service on pressure injury prevention using new research findings. This demonstrates:

A. Evidence dissemination

B. Role delegation
C. Administrative authority
D. Policy enforcement

Q527. A nurse refuses a patient's social media "friend" request to maintain boundaries. This reflects:
A. Empathetic connection
B. Cultural competence
C. Therapeutic communication
D. Professional ethics

Q528. A nurse leader aligns staffing based on patient acuity rather than seniority. This demonstrates:
A. Equity
B. Authority
C. Loyalty
D. Stability

Q529. A nurse develops a teaching plan using adult-learning principles. This approach best represents:
A. Andragogy
B. Pedagogy
C. Mentorship
D. Coaching

Q530. A nurse supports a colleague experiencing burnout by facilitating access to counseling resources. This demonstrates:
A. Compassionate leadership
B. Task management
C. Performance evaluation
D. Disciplinary intervention

Q531. A nurse advocates for including patient satisfaction metrics in performance reviews. This action reflects:
A. Passive observation
B. Hierarchical control
C. Task-centered leadership
D. Quality-focused practice

Q532. A nurse ensures team members understand delegation rules before assigning tasks. This shows:
A. Legal responsibility
B. Ethical neutrality
C. Emotional awareness
D. Passive management

Q533. During interdisciplinary rounds, a nurse clarifies patient goals for consistent care. This exemplifies:
A. Coordination of care
B. Compliance enforcement
C. Role expansion
D. Task repetition

Q534. A nurse promotes shared decision-making with a competent patient refusing a procedure. This supports:
A. Autonomy
B. Beneficence
C. Fidelity
D. Paternalism

Q535. A nurse presents an incident report to risk management after a medication error. This primarily supports:
A. Legal defense
B. Blame assignment
C. Disciplinary review
D. System improvement
Q536. A new nurse expresses uncertainty about delegation tasks. The manager arranges a mentorship. This promotes:
A. Professional development
B. Punitive correction
C. Administrative control
D. Independent practice
Q537. A nurse advocates for bilingual signage in the emergency department. This supports:
A. Health equity
B. Fiscal responsibility
C. Policy compliance
D. Staffing efficiency
Q538. A nurse leader uses feedback from patient surveys to redesign care delivery. This demonstrates:
A. Evidence-informed improvement
B. Top-down leadership
C. Punitive evaluation
D. Task redistribution
Q539. A nurse educator evaluates a training program's outcomes using post-course assessments. This action reflects:
A. Reinforcement stage
B. Planning phase of instruction
C. Implementation phase
D. Evaluation phase of teaching
Q540. A nurse maintains current licensure and fulfills continuing education requirements. This demonstrates:
A. Professional responsibility
B. Administrative compliance
C. External motivation
D. Routine obligation
Q541. A nurse researcher ensures participants voluntarily consent before joining a study. This upholds which ethical principle?
A. Autonomy
B. Justice
C. Beneficence
D. Fidelity
Q542. A nurse participates in a community blood-pressure screening event. This best demonstrates:
A. Health promotion
B. Illness management
C. Risk avoidance
D. Patient advocacy
Q543. A charge nurse handles a staff conflict by encouraging open discussion and mutual problem-solving. This approach reflects:
A. Bureaucratic control

B. Authoritarian supervision
C. Passive management
D. Collaborative leadership

Q544. A nurse uses hospital data to evaluate post-surgery infection rates and suggests changes. This exemplifies:
A. Clinical inquiry
B. Delegation
C. Advocacy
D. Chain of command

Q545. A nurse documents a patient fall accurately and promptly without altering details. This behavior reflects:
A. Integrity
B. Accountability
C. Confidentiality
D. Advocacy

Q546. A nurse leader schedules regular peer review meetings to discuss case outcomes. This strategy primarily supports:
A. Professional growth
B. Financial control
C. Policy enforcement
D. Administrative hierarchy

Q547. A nurse preceptor encourages new graduates to question unclear orders. This approach promotes:
A. Overconfidence
B. Blind obedience
C. Passive compliance
D. Critical thinking

Q548. A nurse helps develop a diversity training program for staff. This supports which professional role component?
A. Cultural competence
B. Legal accountability
C. Task delegation
D. Clinical specialization

Q549. A nurse intervenes when another staff member posts patient information online. This response upholds:
A. Confidentiality
B. Justice
C. Autonomy
D. Fidelity

Q550. A nurse manager evaluates staff retention after implementing flexible scheduling. This reflects:
A. Outcome evaluation
B. Task distribution
C. Policy enforcement
D. Workflow analysis

Q551. A nurse questions a new policy that may jeopardize patient safety. This best demonstrates:
A. Policy resistance
B. Chain of command
C. Procedural compliance

D. Ethical courage

Q552. A nurse documents patient refusal of treatment and notifies the provider. This demonstrates:

A. Respect for autonomy
B. Beneficence
C. Justice
D. Paternalism

Q553. A nurse prepares an evidence-based poster for a professional conference. This activity supports:

A. Knowledge dissemination
B. Direct patient advocacy
C. Operational policy
D. Quality control

Q554. A nurse verifies that informed consent is signed before surgery. This demonstrates:

A. Legal accountability
B. Emotional support
C. Team collaboration
D. Role delegation

Q555. A nurse implements a new pain management protocol validated by recent studies. This is an example of:

A. Experimental research
B. Routine care
C. Protocol adherence
D. Evidence-based practice

Q556. A nurse discusses patient care openly in an elevator. This violates:

A. Confidentiality
B. Accountability
C. Autonomy
D. Fidelity

Q557. A nurse adjusts communication methods to match a patient's literacy level. This reflects:

A. Patient-centered communication
B. Cultural neutrality
C. Time efficiency
D. Standardization

Q558. A nurse joins a professional organization to stay updated on legislative issues. This demonstrates:

A. Professional engagement
B. Political activism
C. Administrative obligation
D. Ethical neutrality

Q559. A nurse documents patient education including understanding and response. This demonstrates:

A. Autonomy
B. Empathy
C. Leadership
D. Accountability

Q560. A nurse ensures continuity of care during shift handoff using SBAR format. This exemplifies:

A. Effective communication
B. Data collection
C. Documentation review

D. Role delegation

Q561. A nurse assists a peer in reflecting on a clinical mistake to identify learning points. This represents:

A. Reflective practice
B. Blame culture
C. Punitive supervision
D. Emotional distancing

Q562. A nurse incorporates hospital ethics guidelines into decision-making. This action shows:

A. Ethical competence
B. Legal liability
C. Administrative obedience
D. Professional neutrality

Q563. A nurse researcher protects subjects by securing data files with encrypted passwords. This supports:

A. Autonomy
B. Beneficence
C. Fidelity
D. Confidentiality

Q564. A nurse leader recognizes team burnout and organizes mindfulness sessions. This illustrates:

A. Supportive leadership
B. Authoritarian style
C. Task management
D. Hierarchical control

Q565. A nurse documents patient care truthfully even when outcomes are unfavorable. This action demonstrates:

A. Integrity
B. Advocacy
C. Objectivity
D. Responsibility

Q566. A nurse uses interprofessional rounds to coordinate discharge planning. This demonstrates:

A. Collaborative practice
B. Administrative leadership
C. Delegation
D. Compliance

Q567. A nurse reports a colleague's repeated lateness affecting patient care. This reflects:

A. Hierarchy
B. Loyalty
C. Conflict avoidance
D. Accountability

Q568. A nurse joins a committee to evaluate ethical dilemmas in end-of-life care. This role emphasizes:

A. Ethical decision-making
B. Resource management
C. Policy enforcement
D. Legal consultation

Q569. A nurse manager promotes transparent communication during incident reviews. This supports:

A. Just culture
B. Punitive policy
C. Defensive documentation

D. Chain-of-command escalation

Q570. A nurse provides an in-service on professional boundaries and social media conduct. This targets:

A. Ethical practice
B. Delegation skills
C. Research literacy
D. Cultural awareness

Q571. A nurse asks a patient's permission before sharing care details with family. This demonstrates:

A. Nonmaleficence
B. Justice
C. Accountability
D. Respect for autonomy

Q572. A nurse leader uses motivational interviewing to encourage adherence to new safety protocols. This reflects:

A. Transformational leadership
B. Transactional supervision
C. Authoritarian style
D. Passive management

Q573. A nurse participates in continuing education to improve cardiac assessment skills. This supports:

A. Lifelong learning
B. Time management
C. Policy enforcement
D. Task delegation

Q574. A nurse manager advocates for improved nurse-patient ratios. This primarily supports:

A. Patient safety
B. Administrative compliance
C. Staffing convenience
D. Fiscal neutrality

Q575. A nurse contributes to updating the unit's orientation manual. This represents:

A. Task distribution
B. Policy enforcement
C. Role delegation
D. Quality improvement

Q576. A nurse engages in self-evaluation to identify performance gaps. This behavior reflects:

A. Reflective practice
B. External audit
C. Peer review
D. Mandatory reporting

Q577. A nurse explains treatment risks clearly before obtaining patient consent. This action reflects:

A. Veracity
B. Beneficence
C. Fidelity
D. Justice

Q578. A nurse educator incorporates simulation to evaluate students' clinical judgment. This demonstrates:

A. Competency-based education
B. Theoretical instruction
C. Research design

D. Policy enforcement

Q579. A nurse volunteers in a disaster-relief mission. This illustrates:

A. Paid service
B. Workplace obligation
C. Policy compliance
D. Professional altruism

Q580. A nurse reports observed discrimination against a coworker. This upholds which professional value?

A. Justice
B. Fidelity
C. Autonomy
D. Confidentiality

Q581. A nurse ensures all team members follow infection-control protocols equally. This demonstrates:

A. Justice
B. Accountability
C. Veracity
D. Advocacy

Q582. A nurse leader acknowledges staff achievements during team meetings. This exemplifies:

A. Positive reinforcement
B. Transactional management
C. Bureaucratic supervision
D. Punitive control

Q583. A nurse participates in a journal club to critique recent research. This best represents:

A. Administrative compliance
B. Routine documentation
C. Mandatory reporting
D. Evidence-based learning

Q584. A nurse explains a medication side effect that was omitted by the provider. This upholds:

A. Veracity
B. Justice
C. Beneficence
D. Fidelity

Q585. A nurse contributes feedback to a new electronic health record (EHR) system rollout. This reflects:

A. Participatory decision-making
B. Hierarchical control
C. Passive observation
D. Administrative compliance

Q586. A nurse supervisor educates staff on proper chain-of-command reporting. This ensures:

A. Structured communication
B. Peer accountability
C. Emotional safety
D. Ethical neutrality

Q587. A nurse manager includes staff nurses in annual goal-setting meetings. This leadership style demonstrates:

A. Transactional leadership
B. Autocratic control

C. Laissez-faire management
D. Democratic leadership

Q588. A nurse counsels a colleague showing signs of compassion fatigue. This demonstrates:
A. Peer support
B. Task supervision
C. Role delegation
D. Administrative control

Q589. A nurse maintains patient records in secure electronic files. This action reflects:
A. Confidentiality
B. Autonomy
C. Justice
D. Fidelity

Q590. A nurse leader collects feedback before implementing a unit-wide scheduling change. This exemplifies:
A. Collaborative management
B. Authoritarian decision-making
C. Passive leadership
D. Delegation

Q591. A nurse reviews institutional policies before performing a new clinical skill. This reflects:
A. Advocacy
B. Empathy
C. Innovation
D. Legal accountability

Q592. A nurse promotes use of interpreter services for non-English-speaking patients. This demonstrates:
A. Cultural competence
B. Fiscal efficiency
C. Role autonomy
D. Policy enforcement

Q593. A nurse expresses concern about unsafe overtime practices affecting patient care. This is an example of:
A. Advocacy
B. Loyalty
C. Resistance
D. Accountability

Q594. A nurse participates in multidisciplinary rounds to plan discharge care. This role supports:
A. Continuity of care
B. Data analysis
C. Task delegation
D. Autonomy

Q595. A nurse apologizes sincerely after a communication misunderstanding with a patient. This demonstrates:
A. Paternalism
B. Legal compliance
C. Emotional detachment
D. Professional accountability

Q596. A nurse encourages new graduates to join professional organizations. This action supports:
A. Professional development

B. Administrative control
C. Routine compliance
D. Peer competition

Q597. A nurse attends a hospital committee to discuss policy updates. This represents:
A. Shared governance
B. Delegation
C. Mentorship
D. Supervision

Q598. A nurse evaluates peer performance using objective criteria during annual review. This ensures:
A. Fair evaluation
B. Personal bias
C. Informal feedback
D. Hierarchical favoritism

Q599. A nurse reviews current literature before updating wound-care guidelines. This activity demonstrates:
A. Compliance
B. Task repetition
C. Delegation
D. Evidence integration

Q600. A nurse reports suspected elder abuse to social services. This demonstrates:
A. Legal and ethical duty
B. Cultural bias
C. Administrative discretion
D. Confidentiality breach

Answer key and Explanation (501-600)

Q501. Answer: B

Explanation: Transformational leaders inspire nurses to integrate evidence-based changes that improve outcomes. Unlike transactional leaders who focus on tasks and rewards, transformational leaders foster innovation and shared vision. Laissez-faire and autocratic styles discourage collaboration and professional growth, reducing team engagement and clinical quality.

Q502. Answer: A

Explanation: Promoting open discussion of near-misses supports a blame-free safety culture that emphasizes learning over punishment. This differs from punitive or hierarchical environments that suppress reporting. Authoritarian supervision limits communication, whereas a just culture encourages transparency and continuous improvement for patient safety.

Q503. Answer: A

Explanation: Mentorship exemplifies collegiality—supporting peers through shared learning and cooperation. Accountability and autonomy relate to individual responsibility and decision-making, not guidance. Confidentiality focuses on protecting patient information, not professional development. Mentoring builds confidence and strengthens clinical competence within the nursing team.

Q504. Answer: B

Explanation: Integrity requires nurses to document truthfully and avoid misrepresentation. It differs from advocacy, which protects patient interests, and beneficence, which promotes well-being. Teamwork involves collaboration but not falsifying records. Upholding integrity maintains ethical standards and legal accountability in nursing documentation.

Q505. Answer: A

Explanation: Advocacy requires speaking up to protect patient safety, such as reporting inadequate staffing. Delegation and paperwork are managerial tasks, not advocacy. Silent compliance may allow unsafe conditions to persist. True advocacy prioritizes patient welfare and ethical responsibility over convenience or hierarchy.

Q506. Answer: A

Explanation: Professional accountability means maintaining competence and applying current policies for safe care. Cultural awareness and empathy relate to interpersonal sensitivity, not adherence to standards. Delegation involves task distribution. Accountability ensures nurses stay informed and uphold institutional safety practices.

Q507. Answer: D

Explanation: Confidentiality protects participant identity and privacy in research. It differs from veracity (truthfulness), justice (fairness), and fidelity (faithfulness to commitments). Maintaining confidentiality sustains trust, encourages honest participation, and fulfills professional ethical obligations in research practice.

Q508. Answer: A

Explanation: Quality improvement focuses on addressing performance gaps to enhance patient outcomes. It differs from cost-driven or punitive approaches. Administrative control enforces policy without development focus. Providing workshops promotes evidence-based competence and continuous professional growth.

Q509. Answer: A

Explanation: Upholding professional boundaries protects patients and nurses by ensuring tasks match legal scope. Refusal differs from negligence or poor teamwork; it safeguards safety and ethics. Over-delegation describes inappropriate task assignment by supervisors, not refusal of unsafe tasks.

Q510. Answer: A

Explanation: Collaboration involves open communication and mutual respect among disciplines. It contrasts with conflict avoidance or hierarchy, which impede shared decision-making. Assertiveness supports collaboration but is one skill within it. True collaboration enhances patient outcomes through integrated expertise.

Q511. Answer: A

Explanation: Measuring hand-hygiene compliance evaluates clinical outcomes and safety metrics. Peer review involves colleague evaluation; self-assessment is individual reflection; and audits are broader system reviews. Outcome measurement supports evidence-based management of infection control performance.

Q512. Answer: B

Explanation: Ethics committee participation reflects advocacy—ensuring patients' rights and ethical care decisions. Educators focus on knowledge transfer; policy developers craft administrative frameworks; researchers generate evidence. Advocacy ensures ethical principles guide institutional practices and patient protections.

Q513. Answer: A

Explanation: Respecting autonomy means supporting informed choice without coercion. Nonmaleficence focuses on avoiding harm, fidelity on keeping promises, and justice on fairness. Facilitating unbiased decision-making empowers patients to participate actively in their care.

Q514. Answer: B

Explanation: Timely documentation maintains accuracy and continuity of care. Delayed or delegated charting increases errors and violates accountability standards. Physician review doesn't replace nursing responsibility. Immediate, factual documentation reflects integrity and professional reliability.

Q515. Answer: B

Explanation: Protecting patient information fulfills confidentiality obligations under HIPAA and nursing ethics. Justice involves fairness; autonomy relates to patient decision-making; veracity concerns truthfulness. Confidentiality maintains trust and legal compliance in professional practice.

Q516. Answer: A

Explanation: A just culture fosters open reporting of errors to improve systems rather than blame individuals. Bureaucratic control and vertical communication discourage openness. Defensive practice leads to fear-based behavior. Just culture enhances learning and organizational safety.

Q517. Answer: A

Explanation: Lifelong learning sustains professional competence and adapts practice to current standards. It differs from time management or supervision, which involve organizational skills. Productivity measures output, not learning. Ongoing education ensures quality and evidence-based care.

Q518. Answer: A

Explanation: Safe delegation ensures the task is appropriate, the delegatee competent, and supervision provided. Abdication means neglecting responsibility, not appropriate delegation. Passive management and avoidance reflect poor leadership. Effective delegation maintains safety and workflow efficiency.

Q519. Answer: A

Explanation: Veracity requires truthfulness even under pressure. Advocacy protects patients; justice ensures fairness; accountability involves owning one's duties. Honest testimony sustains professional integrity and legal credibility within nursing ethics.

Q520. Answer: C

Explanation: Using empirical data to redesign care processes reflects evidence-based practice—integrating research, expertise, and patient needs. Routine procedure and compliance lack analytical evaluation. Intuition alone isn't evidence-driven. Data-guided improvement enhances quality and outcomes.

Q521. Answer: A

Explanation: Shared governance empowers nurses to contribute to policy development and decision-making, enhancing professional ownership. Delegation focuses on task distribution, advocacy on patient rights, and case management on care coordination. Shared governance strengthens collaboration and improves institutional standards through staff engagement.

Q522. Answer: B

Explanation: Therapeutic communication fosters understanding and emotional support through empathy and clarity. Cultural competence includes sensitivity to diverse beliefs but is broader. Passive listening lacks feedback, and technical accuracy alone omits compassion. Effective communication enhances trust and shared decision-making.

Q523. Answer: C

Explanation: Accountability involves upholding professional standards and protecting patient safety, even when reporting peers. Fidelity refers to loyalty, justice to fairness, and beneficence to doing good. Reporting misconduct preserves integrity and ensures safe, ethical care for patients and colleagues.

Q524. Answer: A

Explanation: Democratic leaders value team input and collective decision-making, fostering engagement and innovation. Autocratic leaders make unilateral decisions, transactional leaders emphasize performance and reward, and laissez-faire leaders provide minimal direction. Democratic leadership enhances morale and professional accountability.

Q525. Answer: A

Explanation: Cultural humility involves open, respectful exploration of patient beliefs to provide inclusive care. Correcting or avoiding discussions limits trust. Rejecting rituals without understanding disrespects diversity. Humility fosters patient-centered care aligned with cultural and ethical principles.

Q526. Answer: A

Explanation: Sharing current research findings promotes evidence dissemination, bridging the gap between knowledge and practice. Delegation and authority involve management, not education. Policy enforcement applies existing rules, while dissemination actively updates colleagues to improve outcomes and professional growth.

Q527. Answer: D

Explanation: Declining social media contact preserves professional ethics and protects confidentiality. While communication and empathy are important, boundary maintenance prevents conflicts of interest. Cultural competence concerns respect for beliefs, not online behavior. Ethical conduct ensures professionalism and trust.

Q528. Answer: A

Explanation: Equity ensures fair resource allocation according to need, not hierarchy. Authority and loyalty relate to power and allegiance, not fairness. Stability addresses consistency, not appropriateness. Equity supports patient safety and workload balance through objective staffing decisions.

Q529. Answer: A

Explanation: Andragogy emphasizes self-directed, experience-based learning suited for adults. Pedagogy applies to dependent learners. Mentorship and coaching are relational processes within teaching but not the underlying learning theory. Applying andragogy promotes engagement and knowledge retention among adult nurses.

Q530. Answer: A

Explanation: Compassionate leadership prioritizes empathy, emotional well-being, and supportive action. Task management and evaluation focus on operations, not emotional care. Disciplinary measures are punitive. Compassionate leadership fosters resilience and a positive professional culture.

Q531. Answer: D

Explanation: Integrating patient satisfaction emphasizes continuous quality improvement and outcome accountability.y. Hierarchical control limits participation, task-centered leadership ignores holistic care, and passive observation lacks engagement. Quality-focused practice prioritizes measurable, patient-centered standards for professional evaluation.

Q532. Answer: A
Explanation: Delegation within scope demonstrates legal responsibility and compliance with the Nurse Practice Act. Ethical neutrality implies indecision, and emotional awareness concerns interpersonal dynamics. Passive management avoids accountability. Understanding delegation law ensures safety and liability protection.
Q533. Answer: A
Explanation: Coordinating care ensures team alignment on patient goals, avoiding duplication and confusion. Compliance enforcement enforces rules, not collaboration. Role expansion describes assuming new responsibilities, and task repetition lacks coordination focus. Collaboration strengthens continuity and efficiency in multidisciplinary care.
Q534. Answer: A
Explanation: Respecting autonomy honors patients' right to make informed choices, even if they differ from recommendations. Beneficence promotes welfare but may conflict with autonomy. Fidelity ensures loyalty, and paternalism overrides choice. Upholding autonomy maintains ethical integrity and trust.
Q535. Answer: D
Explanation: Reporting errors supports system improvement and prevention, not punishment. Blame or disciplinary review undermines safety culture. Legal defense is secondary to learning. Transparent reporting identifies root causes and enhances patient safety outcomes.
Q536. Answer: A
Explanation: Mentorship builds confidence and skill through guidance, supporting professional growth. Punitive or administrative actions discourage learning. Independent practice without mentorship risks errors. Structured mentorship fosters competence and retention.
Q537. Answer: A
Explanation: Providing multilingual resources ensures health equity by improving access and understanding for diverse populations. Fiscal responsibility and compliance address finances and regulations, not fairness. Equity-driven advocacy promotes inclusion and patient-centered care.
Q538. Answer: A
Explanation: Integrating patient feedback into practice changes reflects evidence-informed improvement—combining data and clinical expertise. Top-down or punitive approaches discourage engagement. Task redistribution focuses on workload, not quality. Evidence use enhances satisfaction and outcomes.
Q539. Answer: D
Explanation: Evaluation measures learning effectiveness and guides future improvements. Planning sets goals, implementation delivers content, and reinforcement strengthens retention. Evaluation ensures accountability and continuous improvement in education.
Q540. Answer: A
Explanation: Maintaining licensure and education reflects professional responsibility—commitment to competence and ethical practice. Administrative compliance is external, while true professionalism is self-motivated. Routine obligation lacks engagement. Responsibility ensures credibility and safe patient care.
Q541. Answer: A
Explanation: Autonomy involves respecting individuals' rights to make informed, voluntary choices. Justice ensures fairness, beneficence promotes good, and fidelity concerns loyalty. Obtaining consent honors autonomy by protecting participants from coercion and maintaining ethical research integrity.
Q542. Answer: A
Explanation: Health promotion focuses on preventing disease and improving wellness in populations. Illness management begins after diagnosis, and risk avoidance is a subset of prevention. Advocacy

supports patient rights, not proactive outreach. Community screenings enhance prevention and early detection.

Q543. Answer: D

Explanation: Collaborative leadership resolves conflict through open communication and shared decision-making. Authoritarian and bureaucratic styles restrict dialogue, while passive management avoids resolution. Collaboration promotes trust, engagement, and sustainable team relationships.

Q544. Answer: A

Explanation: Clinical inquiry applies data and research methods to improve care. Delegation assigns duties, not analysis. Advocacy protects patients but doesn't analyze outcomes. Chain of command ensures reporting structure, not quality evaluation. Inquiry drives evidence-based improvement.

Q545. Answer: A

Explanation: Integrity means honesty and accuracy in documentation, even when incidents occur. Accountability involves accepting responsibility, but integrity emphasizes truthfulness. Confidentiality protects privacy, and advocacy promotes patient rights. Integrity ensures legal and ethical reliability of clinical records.

Q546. Answer: A

Explanation: Peer review fosters learning, feedback, and quality improvement through professional dialogue. It differs from financial or administrative controls. Policy enforcement ensures compliance, not learning. Structured peer feedback strengthens clinical judgment and evidence-based performance.

Q547. Answer: D

Explanation: Encouraging questioning builds critical thinking and safety awareness. Blind obedience and passive compliance risk errors. Overconfidence without inquiry leads to mistakes. Critical thinking ensures nurses assess information logically before action, reinforcing safe practice.

Q548. Answer: A

Explanation: Promoting diversity awareness enhances cultural competence—understanding and valuing patient and staff differences. Legal accountability ensures compliance but doesn't address inclusion. Delegation and specialization relate to tasks or roles, not cultural understanding. Cultural competence improves patient satisfaction and equity.

Q549. Answer: A

Explanation: Protecting patient information maintains confidentiality, a legal and ethical duty. Justice relates to fairness, autonomy to personal choice, and fidelity to loyalty. Breaches of confidentiality erode trust and violate HIPAA and professional standards.

Q550. Answer: A

Explanation: Assessing retention measures outcomes related to staff satisfaction and organizational performance. Task distribution and workflow analysis manage operations, while policy enforcement ensures compliance. Outcome evaluation connects management strategies with measurable improvements.

Q551. Answer: D

Explanation: Ethical courage involves voicing safety concerns despite potential conflict. Using the chain of command is procedural, while compliance and resistance lack ethical motivation. Courage supports advocacy and integrity, prioritizing patient welfare over conformity.

Q552. Answer: A

Explanation: Respecting autonomy means honoring a competent patient's decision to decline care. Beneficence promotes welfare, and justice ensures fairness, but autonomy governs self-determination. Paternalism overrides choice. Documentation and communication safeguard patient rights and legal accountability.

Q553. Answer: A

Explanation: Presenting research findings promotes knowledge dissemination, advancing professional standards. Advocacy focuses on patient rights, and policy or quality control address administration. Sharing evidence fosters innovation and peer learning across the nursing profession.

Q554. Answer: A

Explanation: Ensuring informed consent upholds legal accountability and patient rights. Emotional support provides reassurance but not legal compliance. Collaboration and delegation are teamwork concepts, not consent verification. Legal vigilance safeguards patient autonomy and institutional integrity.

Q555. Answer: D

Explanation: Evidence-based practice integrates research, expertise, and patient preferences into care. Routine or protocol adherence may lack current validation. Experimental research tests hypotheses, not application. Evidence use ensures clinical effectiveness and best outcomes.

Q556. Answer: A

Explanation: Discussing patient details publicly breaches confidentiality, violating HIPAA and ethical standards. Accountability relates to responsibility, autonomy to decision-making, and fidelity to loyalty. Protecting privacy is essential to professional trust and patient rights.

Q557. Answer: A

Explanation: Tailoring communication ensures understanding and empowerment—key elements of patient-centered care. Cultural neutrality ignores individual needs, and time efficiency focuses on speed. Standardization limits personalization. Effective communication improves compliance and outcomes.

Q558. Answer: A

Explanation: Joining organizations fosters professional engagement and awareness of evolving standards. Political activism is more advocacy-driven; obligation and neutrality lack initiative. Active involvement supports lifelong learning and influence in policy shaping.

Q559. Answer: D

Explanation: Documentation of teaching outcomes confirms accountability for communication and comprehension. Empathy and leadership enhance interaction but aren't record-keeping duties. Autonomy involves decision-making. Accountability ensures continuity, safety, and legal completeness.

Q560. Answer: A

Explanation: SBAR ensures structured, effective communication for safe transitions. Data collection and documentation review support communication but aren't the exchange itself. Delegation assigns tasks. SBAR standardizes clarity, reducing errors and enhancing teamwork.

Q561. Answer: A

Explanation: Reflective practice encourages self-analysis for growth and prevention of future errors. Unlike blame or punitive culture, it promotes learning and resilience. Emotional distancing avoids engagement. Reflection strengthens accountability and continuous improvement in nursing performance.

Q562. Answer: A

Explanation: Ethical competence involves integrating moral frameworks into daily practice. Legal liability concerns compliance, not values. Obedience and neutrality reflect passive behavior. Ethical competence ensures nurses balance principles like justice, beneficence, and autonomy in care delivery.

Q563. Answer: D

Explanation: Protecting data ensures confidentiality and respects participants' privacy. Beneficence promotes welfare, fidelity means loyalty, and autonomy governs decision-making. Data security upholds trust and meets ethical research requirements for information protection.

Q564. Answer: A

Explanation: Supportive leadership prioritizes staff well-being, preventing burnout and fostering engagement. Authoritarian and hierarchical styles focus on authority rather than empathy. Task management organizes duties but doesn't address morale. Supportive leadership sustains retention and productivity.

Q565. Answer: A

Explanation: Integrity ensures honesty regardless of result, preserving ethical and legal credibility. Advocacy defends patient rights, objectivity avoids bias, and responsibility implies duty. Integrity reinforces transparency and trustworthiness in nursing documentation.

Q566. Answer: A

Explanation: Collaborative practice unites multiple disciplines for seamless care. Administrative leadership focuses on management, delegation assigns tasks, and compliance enforces policy. Collaboration enhances communication and continuity during transitions, improving patient outcomes and team efficiency.

Q567. Answer: D

Explanation: Accountability requires addressing issues compromising patient safety or team function. Loyalty cannot override professional duty. Avoiding conflict perpetuates problems, and hierarchy concerns authority structure. Accountability maintains standards and reliability in healthcare teams.

Q568. Answer: A

Explanation: Serving on an ethics committee fosters ethical decision-making, balancing principles like autonomy, beneficence, and justice. Resource or policy roles lack moral analysis focus. Legal consultation provides technical advice, not value deliberation. Ethical input ensures humane, principled care.

Q569. Answer: A

Explanation: A just culture encourages openness and learning from errors without undue blame. Punitive and defensive approaches suppress honesty. Chain escalation manages hierarchy, not safety learning. Just culture enhances trust and continuous system improvement.

Q570. Answer: A

Explanation: Educating peers on social media boundaries reinforces ethical practice and confidentiality. Delegation and research skills are technical, while cultural awareness focuses on diversity. Ethics education ensures professionalism and safeguards patient trust in digital communication.

Q571. Answer: D

Explanation: Obtaining consent respects autonomy and privacy. Justice ensures fairness, accountability manages responsibility, and nonmaleficence avoids harm. Honoring patient consent reflects ethical communication and confidentiality.

Q572. Answer: A

Explanation: Transformational leaders motivate through dialogue and shared purpose. Transactional leaders rely on rewards, authoritarian ones enforce commands, and passive managers disengage. Transformational leadership fosters empowerment and ownership in safety initiatives.

Q573. Answer: A

Explanation: Lifelong learning sustains competence and evidence-based practice. Time management and policy enforcement are operational. Delegation involves task assignment, not education. Ongoing learning ensures clinical excellence and adaptation to current standards.

Q574. Answer: A

Explanation: Advocating for safe ratios protects patient outcomes and reduces nurse fatigue. Compliance and fiscal neutrality prioritize budget over safety. Advocacy ensures ethical care quality and staff well-being through equitable workloads.

Q575. Answer: D

Explanation: Revising manuals enhances quality improvement by standardizing evidence-based procedures. Enforcement and delegation apply after development. Updating ensures accuracy, consistency, and effective onboarding aligned with professional standards.

Q576. Answer: A

Explanation: Reflective practice promotes self-assessment and continual growth. External audits and peer reviews involve others' evaluations, while mandatory reporting addresses compliance. Reflection builds insight and fosters self-directed professional development.

Q577. Answer: A

Explanation: Veracity requires honesty and full disclosure to support informed decisions. Beneficence promotes welfare, fidelity ensures faithfulness, and justice focuses on fairness. Truthful communication underpins ethical, patient-centered care.

Q578. Answer: A

Explanation: Simulation assesses competency by applying knowledge in realistic scenarios. Theoretical teaching focuses on concepts, research design collects data, and policy enforcement manages rules. Competency-based education bridges theory and practice effectively.

Q579. Answer: D

Explanation: Volunteering for humanitarian aid exemplifies altruism—selfless service beyond duty. Obligation and compliance imply requirement, while paid service lacks voluntary motivation. Altruism reflects compassion and professional commitment to community welfare.

Q580. Answer: A

Explanation: Justice ensures fairness and equal treatment in professional environments. Fidelity means loyalty, autonomy governs self-determination, and confidentiality protects information. Reporting bias demonstrates ethical integrity and advocacy for equitable workplace culture.

Q581. Answer: A

Explanation: Justice ensures fair treatment and consistent adherence to safety standards. Accountability involves personal responsibility, veracity focuses on truth, and advocacy defends patient rights. Equal protocol enforcement supports ethical fairness and safe patient environments.

Q582. Answer: A

Explanation: Positive reinforcement motivates employees by recognizing accomplishments and encouraging continued excellence. Transactional and bureaucratic management rely on rules and rewards, while punitive control discourages morale. Recognition enhances engagement and fosters a supportive culture.

Q583. Answer: D

Explanation: Discussing research fosters evidence-based learning and critical appraisal skills. Documentation, reporting, and compliance are procedural, not analytical. Engaging with literature promotes informed decision-making and professional growth.

Q584. Answer: A

Explanation: Veracity requires truthfulness to ensure patients make fully informed decisions. Justice ensures fairness, beneficence promotes good, and fidelity implies loyalty. Providing complete information preserves ethical transparency and patient trust.

Q585. Answer: A

Explanation: Participatory decision-making engages staff in evaluating and improving systems they use. Hierarchy and compliance impose top-down control, while passive observation lacks initiative. Involvement improves usability and promotes ownership of organizational change.

Q586. Answer: A

Explanation: Chain-of-command protocols maintain structured, transparent communication for timely issue resolution. Peer accountability is interpersonal, emotional safety supports culture, and neutrality avoids ethical engagement. Proper structure minimizes risk and enhances clarity in operations.

Q587. Answer: D

Explanation: Democratic leaders promote inclusion and shared governance, enhancing motivation and innovation. Autocratic and transactional styles focus on authority or reward systems, while laissez-faire lacks direction. Inclusion strengthens teamwork and organizational alignment.

Q588. Answer: A
Explanation: Peer support fosters well-being and resilience through empathy and listening. Task supervision manages performance, not emotions. Delegation and control address workflow, not morale. Supportive interactions maintain mental health and collegial trust.
Q589. Answer: A
Explanation: Confidentiality ensures patient data privacy and legal compliance under HIPAA. Autonomy relates to choice, justice to fairness, and fidelity to loyalty. Protecting records safeguards trust and upholds ethical nursing practice.
Q590. Answer: A
Explanation: Collaborative management values team input for effective change. Authoritarian and passive leadership ignore participation. Delegation assigns tasks, not governance. Collaboration builds consensus and fosters staff satisfaction in decision processes.
Q591. Answer: D
Explanation: Checking policies ensures legal and professional accountability for safe, compliant practice. Empathy relates to emotional care, innovation to creativity, and advocacy to rights protection. Legal awareness prevents errors and liability.
Q592. Answer: A
Explanation: Providing interpreters ensures cultural competence and equitable communication. Fiscal efficiency and autonomy may conflict with access needs. Policy enforcement ensures rules but not sensitivity. Cultural competence enhances safety and patient satisfaction.
Q593. Answer: A
Explanation: Advocacy defends patient and staff welfare by identifying unsafe practices. Loyalty prioritizes individuals, resistance implies opposition without purpose, and accountability means personal duty. Advocacy drives ethical improvement and safety.
Q594. Answer: A
Explanation: Participation ensures coordinated, continuous care across disciplines. Data analysis examines outcomes, delegation assigns tasks, and autonomy applies to independence. Collaboration ensures safe transitions and patient-centered planning.
Q595. Answer: D
Explanation: Apologizing acknowledges accountability, preserving trust and professionalism. Compliance focuses on regulations, detachment reduces empathy, and paternalism overrides patient input. Accountability strengthens relationships through transparency and respect.
Q596. Answer: A
Explanation: Joining organizations promotes professional development, networking, and leadership growth. Control and compliance imply obligation, and competition fosters rivalry. Professional engagement enhances career progression and shared learning.
Q597. Answer: A
Explanation: Shared governance allows staff input in institutional decisions, empowering nurses. Delegation and supervision manage workflow, not policy. Mentorship guides individuals, not governance. Participation fosters ownership and accountability.
Q598. Answer: A
Explanation: Using objective criteria supports fairness and transparency. Bias and favoritism undermine credibility, while informal feedback lacks structure. Fair evaluation builds trust and motivates professional growth.
Q599. Answer: D
Explanation: Reviewing research ensures evidence integration into clinical standards. Repetition and delegation manage workflow, not knowledge application. Compliance ensures rule following, not innovation. Evidence integration maintains currency and quality in care delivery.

Q600. Answer: A

Explanation: Reporting abuse fulfills legal and ethical responsibilities under mandatory reporting laws. Cultural bias and discretion imply judgment or avoidance. Confidentiality does not prevent lawful protection measures. Reporting ensures patient safety and justice.

Questions (601-650)

Q601. A nurse ensures fairness when distributing assignments among staff based on patient acuity. This action demonstrates:

A. Justice
B. Accountability
C. Fidelity
D. Veracity

Q602. A nurse manager uses incident reports to develop targeted safety education. This illustrates:

A. Quality improvement
B. Punitive management
C. Administrative reporting
D. Policy enforcement

Q603. A nurse signs a confidentiality agreement before accessing electronic patient records. This reflects:

A. Beneficence
B. Advocacy
C. Legal compliance
D. Team collaboration

Q604. A nurse demonstrates fidelity by:

A. Following through on promised patient care actions
B. Maintaining equal workload distribution
C. Delegating tasks effectively
D. Reporting unsafe staffing levels

Q605. A nurse discloses medication errors promptly to the patient and provider. This upholds:

A. Veracity
B. Confidentiality
C. Loyalty
D. Justice

Q606. A nurse regularly checks professional practice standards to ensure compliance. This represents:

A. Professional accountability
B. Autonomy
C. Cultural competence
D. Advocacy

Q607. A nurse explains research findings to colleagues and encourages their application in practice. This behavior demonstrates:

A. Administrative supervision
B. Delegation
C. Ethical neutrality
D. Evidence dissemination

Q608. A nurse maintains a respectful tone when addressing conflict with a physician. This demonstrates:

A. Professional communication
B. Passive behavior
C. Assertive avoidance
D. Emotional detachment

Q609. A nurse observes a colleague using an expired medication and intervenes immediately. This reflects:

A. Patient advocacy
B. Autonomy
C. Justice
D. Fidelity

Q610. A nurse manager invites staff input before revising unit policies. This reflects:
A. Shared governance
B. Task delegation
C. Administrative authority
D. Policy enforcement

Q611. A nurse discloses financial relationships when participating in clinical research. This demonstrates:
A. Advocacy
B. Autonomy
C. Confidentiality
D. Transparency

Q612. A nurse consistently follows infection-control policies despite time constraints. This best reflects:
A. Professional integrity
B. Task prioritization
C. Compliance pressure
D. Delegation efficiency

Q613. A nurse ensures informed consent includes both risks and benefits of a procedure. This upholds:
A. Autonomy
B. Justice
C. Veracity
D. Beneficence

Q614. A nurse mentor helps new staff set realistic career goals. This demonstrates:
A. Professional development support
B. Administrative control
C. Evaluative supervision
D. Peer delegation

Q615. A nurse advocates for palliative care access for underserved populations. This reflects:
A. Fidelity
B. Beneficence
C. Veracity
D. Social justice

Q616. A nurse leads a debriefing after a critical incident to identify system issues. This illustrates:
A. Reflective leadership
B. Punitive supervision
C. Passive management
D. Authoritarian control

Q617. A nurse upholds confidentiality when discussing a case during teaching rounds. This demonstrates:
A. Ethical conduct
B. Assertiveness
C. Accountability
D. Autonomy

Q618. A nurse educator ensures teaching materials meet literacy standards for diverse learners. This supports:
A. Health literacy
B. Delegation
C. Compliance
D. Efficiency
Q619. A nurse submits data for national benchmarking reports. This action supports:
A. Ethical neutrality
B. Advocacy
C. Quality measurement
D. Emotional support
Q620. A nurse promptly reports a breach in patient data security. This reflects:
A. Legal responsibility
B. Team collaboration
C. Beneficence
D. Autonomy
Q621. A nurse discusses a patient's case privately in a closed meeting room. This behavior upholds:
A. Confidentiality
B. Justice
C. Autonomy
D. Accountability
Q622. A nurse evaluates the effectiveness of pain-management education after discharge. This represents:
A. Outcome evaluation
B. Delegation
C. Policy enforcement
D. Staff education
Q623. A nurse develops a fall-prevention poster using updated evidence. This reflects:
A. Research design
B. Routine procedure
C. Policy compliance
D. Evidence-based practice
Q624. A nurse attends ethics training to strengthen decision-making in complex cases. This supports:
A. Ethical competence
B. Professional hierarchy
C. Clinical delegation
D. Task efficiency
Q625. A nurse addresses a medication discrepancy immediately with the provider. This demonstrates:
A. Patient advocacy
B. Passive communication
C. Administrative compliance
D. Hierarchical obedience
Q626. A nurse documents all interventions objectively, avoiding assumptions. This represents:
A. Accuracy in documentation
B. Empathetic communication
C. Task completion
D. Delegation
Q627. A nurse promotes patient participation in care decisions. This reflects:

A. Fidelity
B. Beneficence
C. Justice
D. Respect for autonomy

Q628. A nurse informs staff about changes to infection-control guidelines based on new evidence. This illustrates:

A. Knowledge translation
B. Policy enforcement
C. Delegation
D. Administrative control

Q629. A nurse manager uses staff surveys to improve morale and retention. This action represents:

A. Employee engagement
B. Punitive management
C. Bureaucratic control
D. Task delegation

Q630. A nurse shares research findings in a unit meeting. This demonstrates:

A. Professional scholarship
B. Chain-of-command adherence
C. Administrative leadership
D. Clinical delegation

Q631. A nurse updates care plans daily to reflect patient progress. This behavior indicates:

A. Autonomy
B. Advocacy
C. Leadership
D. Accountability

Q632. A nurse collaborates with a dietitian to modify a diabetic patient's meal plan. This is an example of:

A. Interprofessional collaboration
B. Task delegation
C. Administrative policy
D. Ethical supervision

Q633. A nurse acts as a preceptor for nursing students. This reflects:

A. Professional mentorship
B. Quality control
C. Policy enforcement
D. Administrative evaluation

Q634. A nurse leader facilitates conflict resolution between two staff members. This demonstrates:

A. Emotional intelligence
B. Task supervision
C. Passive mediation
D. Administrative control

Q635. A nurse conducts a peer review using evidence-based standards. This practice supports:

A. Hierarchical control
B. Personal criticism
C. Informal feedback
D. Professional accountability

Q636. A nurse participates in ethics rounds to discuss patient dilemmas. This activity emphasizes:

A. Reflective ethics practice

B. Policy compliance
C. Delegation efficiency
D. Administrative review

Q637. A nurse explains discharge instructions to ensure patient understanding. This reflects:
A. Patient education
B. Data verification
C. Task repetition
D. Delegation

Q638. A nurse who volunteers for a policy committee on workplace safety demonstrates:
A. Leadership initiative
B. Administrative duty
C. Task assignment
D. Routine compliance

Q639. A nurse promptly reports a near-miss incident to risk management. This supports:
A. Punitive discipline
B. Defensive practice
C. Hierarchical control
D. Safety culture

Q640. A nurse consistently attends staff education sessions and applies new practices. This reflects:
A. Commitment to lifelong learning
B. Administrative compliance
C. Time management
D. Routine obligation

Q641. A nurse advocates for the inclusion of evidence-based pain protocols in hospital policy. This demonstrates:
A. Leadership in practice improvement
B. Task delegation
C. Routine compliance
D. Administrative control

Q642. A nurse leader rewards staff for consistently meeting patient satisfaction goals. This leadership approach reflects:
A. Passive supervision
B. Transformational leadership
C. Autocratic management
D. Transactional leadership

Q643. A nurse participates in data collection for a research study while maintaining objectivity. This reflects:
A. Research integrity
B. Task efficiency
C. Administrative neutrality
D. Policy adherence

Q644. A nurse includes social determinants of health when developing community care plans. This reflects:
A. Holistic practice
B. Cultural bias
C. Administrative focus
D. Legal compliance

Q645. A nurse uses active listening when counseling a distressed family member. This demonstrates:

A. Therapeutic communication
B. Emotional detachment
C. Task prioritization
D. Directive counseling

Q646. A nurse provides factual feedback during a peer performance evaluation. This behavior supports:

A. Emotional support
B. Collegial loyalty
C. Objectivity
D. Conflict avoidance

Q647. A nurse promotes teamwork by acknowledging diverse perspectives during care planning. This demonstrates:

A. Inclusivity
B. Authority
C. Passive leadership
D. Competition

Q648. A nurse notifies the infection-control team about a cluster of postoperative fevers. This reflects:

A. Surveillance responsibility
B. Delegation
C. Chain-of-command escalation
D. Routine compliance

Q649. A nurse recognizes a colleague's exemplary ethical behavior during rounds and shares it in a staff meeting. This supports:

A. Favoritism
B. Administrative promotion
C. Role modeling
D. Passive recognition

Q650. A nurse concludes each shift by evaluating outcomes and identifying learning needs for improvement. This exemplifies:

A. Reflective practice
B. Task review
C. Supervision
D. Administrative evaluation

Answer key and Explanation (601-650)

Q601. Answer: A

Explanation: Justice involves fair, equitable distribution of resources and workload according to need. Accountability ensures responsibility but not fairness. Fidelity relates to loyalty, and veracity means truthfulness. Promoting justice enhances balance, safety, and team morale.

Q602. Answer: A

Explanation: Using data to guide safety education demonstrates quality improvement—transforming incidents into opportunities for learning. Punitive and enforcement approaches discourage openness. Quality improvement promotes continuous system-based prevention and staff competence.

Q603. Answer: C

Explanation: Signing confidentiality agreements fulfills legal and institutional requirements to protect patient information. Advocacy promotes patient rights, while beneficence and collaboration address care quality. Compliance ensures ethical and lawful data management.

Q604. Answer: A

Explanation: Fidelity means keeping promises and maintaining trust with patients. Justice ensures fairness, delegation manages workload, and reporting concerns advocacy. Fulfilling commitments strengthens therapeutic relationships and professional integrity.

Q605. Answer: A

Explanation: Veracity requires honesty and full disclosure to support patient autonomy and safety. Concealing errors breaches ethical transparency. Confidentiality protects privacy but does not override disclosure of harm. Truthful communication reinforces accountability and trust.

Q606. Answer: A

Explanation: Accountability involves maintaining current knowledge and adhering to standards of care. Autonomy emphasizes decision-making, cultural competence focuses on diversity, and advocacy defends rights. Accountability ensures consistency and safe, ethical practice.

Q607. Answer: D

Explanation: Sharing and promoting evidence-based findings improves collective practice. Delegation and supervision distribute tasks, not knowledge. Ethical neutrality avoids engagement. Evidence dissemination promotes learning, innovation, and improved outcomes.

Q608. Answer: A

Explanation: Professional communication balances assertiveness and respect, promoting resolution and collaboration. Passive or avoidant responses suppress dialogue, and detachment impedes teamwork. Effective communication ensures safety and professional relationships.

Q609. Answer: A

Explanation: Advocacy protects patient safety through timely intervention. Autonomy concerns decision rights, justice addresses fairness, and fidelity ensures loyalty. Speaking up ensures harm prevention and adherence to safety standards.

Q610. Answer: A

Explanation: Shared governance promotes participatory leadership and staff ownership. Delegation and authority relate to management tasks, not decision-sharing. Policy enforcement ensures adherence but not collaboration. Involvement increases engagement and innovation.

Q611. Answer: D

Explanation: Transparency ensures honesty and prevents conflicts of interest. Autonomy addresses decision rights, confidentiality protects information, and advocacy defends participants. Openness maintains research credibility and public trust.

Q612. Answer: A

Explanation: Integrity means adhering to ethical and safety standards even when inconvenient. Prioritization organizes tasks, and compliance pressure implies external motivation. Integrity ensures patient safety and professionalism.

Q613. Answer: A

Explanation: Providing full information supports patient autonomy—the right to make informed choices. Justice ensures fairness, veracity ensures honesty, and beneficence promotes welfare. Autonomy emphasizes self-determination through informed decisions.

Q614. Answer: A

Explanation: Mentorship fosters professional growth through guidance and encouragement. Administrative and evaluative roles focus on authority, not development. Delegation assigns tasks, not mentorship. Support strengthens confidence and career progression.

Q615. Answer: D

Explanation: Social justice promotes equitable care for all populations. Beneficence focuses on doing good for individuals, veracity on truthfulness, and fidelity on loyalty. Advocacy for equity embodies nursing's ethical duty to fairness and inclusion.

Q616. Answer: A

Explanation: Reflective leadership encourages learning through open discussion of errors. Punitive or authoritarian responses suppress communication, while passive management avoids engagement. Reflection builds resilience and system improvement.

Q617. Answer: A

Explanation: Ethical conduct ensures patient information is shared only for educational or clinical benefit without violating privacy. Assertiveness and accountability are important but secondary. Ethical care protects rights and maintains professional trust.

Q618. Answer: A

Explanation: Adjusting educational content for comprehension enhances health literacy and patient engagement. Delegation and compliance focus on process, not understanding. Promoting literacy ensures informed care and equitable outcomes.

Q619. Answer: C

Explanation: Benchmarking evaluates performance against standards to improve quality. Advocacy and support serve interpersonal goals, not data analysis. Quality measurement ensures accountability and continuous improvement in healthcare outcomes.

Q620. Answer: A

Explanation: Reporting breaches fulfills legal and ethical duties to protect patient privacy. Collaboration supports teamwork, beneficence promotes welfare, and autonomy relates to choice. Legal responsibility safeguards institutional compliance and trust.

Q621. Answer: A

Explanation: Confidentiality protects patient information by ensuring discussions occur in secure settings. Justice ensures fairness, autonomy supports choice, and accountability ensures responsibility. Maintaining privacy meets ethical and legal standards in professional communication.

Q622. Answer: A

Explanation: Assessing patient understanding and results measures outcome effectiveness. Delegation assigns tasks, policy enforcement ensures compliance, and staff education targets professionals. Outcome evaluation ensures interventions achieve desired learning and clinical impact.

Q623. Answer: D

Explanation: Translating evidence into practical tools demonstrates evidence-based practice. Routine procedures and compliance apply rules without analysis. Research design creates studies but doesn't apply findings. Evidence integration bridges research and bedside care.

Q624. Answer: A

Explanation: Ethics education enhances moral reasoning and professional competence. Hierarchy and delegation address structure, not ethics. Task efficiency improves workflow, not integrity. Ethical competence ensures responsible, principled practice.

Q625. Answer: A

Explanation: Advocacy prioritizes patient safety by clarifying errors. Passive or obedient responses risk harm. Administrative compliance follows policy without initiative. Speaking up ensures ethical and clinical accountability.

Q626. Answer: A

Explanation: Objectivity ensures factual, unbiased documentation critical for legal and clinical accuracy. Empathy aids communication, but records require neutrality. Task completion and delegation involve workflow, not integrity. Accurate records ensure continuity and accountability.

Q627. Answer: D

Explanation: Encouraging involvement supports autonomy—the right to self-determination. Beneficence promotes good, justice ensures fairness, and fidelity upholds loyalty. Empowering patients strengthens trust and collaborative care.

Q628. Answer: A

Explanation: Knowledge translation applies research findings into clinical protocols. Policy enforcement ensures rule adherence, not understanding. Delegation distributes tasks. Translating knowledge improves practice consistency and safety outcomes.

Q629. Answer: A

Explanation: Seeking feedback promotes engagement by addressing workplace satisfaction. Punitive or bureaucratic methods suppress communication, and delegation organizes duties, not morale. Engagement fosters loyalty and collaboration.

Q630. Answer: A

Explanation: Sharing evidence reflects scholarship and commitment to professional development. Chain adherence and leadership focus on structure, not learning. Delegation involves task assignment. Scholarship fosters knowledge growth and peer advancement.

Q631. Answer: D

Explanation: Regularly updating care plans maintains accountability for accuracy and ongoing assessment. Advocacy and leadership involve broader actions, while autonomy governs decision-making. Accountability ensures continuity and quality documentation.

Q632. Answer: A

Explanation: Working with other disciplines exemplifies interprofessional collaboration, enhancing holistic care. Delegation and policy focus on structure, not teamwork. Collaboration improves patient outcomes through shared expertise.

Q633. Answer: A

Explanation: Serving as a preceptor supports mentorship and knowledge transfer. Quality control and enforcement maintain standards, not teaching. Mentorship builds confidence and promotes workforce development.

Q634. Answer: A

Explanation: Emotional intelligence involves empathy, awareness, and mediation to manage conflict constructively. Supervision and control focus on hierarchy, not understanding. Emotional intelligence strengthens teamwork and morale.

Q635. Answer: D

Explanation: Evidence-based peer review fosters accountability and quality improvement. Personal criticism undermines professionalism, while informal or hierarchical reviews lack structure. Accountability promotes fairness and continuous development.

Q636. Answer: A

Explanation: Ethics rounds encourage reflection on moral issues and principles. Policy and administrative reviews focus on rules, not values. Reflection deepens ethical reasoning and teamwork in complex cases.

Q637. Answer: A

Explanation: Providing clear education ensures comprehension and adherence to care plans. Verification and repetition confirm accuracy but don't teach. Education empowers patients and promotes safe recovery.

Q638. Answer: A

Explanation: Volunteering shows leadership initiative and commitment to safety improvement. Administrative duties and routine compliance are mandatory, not voluntary. Initiative drives engagement and systemic progress.

Q639. Answer: D

Explanation: Reporting near misses promotes a safety culture focused on prevention and learning. Defensive or punitive approaches hide errors. Open reporting reduces risks and improves systems.

Q640. Answer: A

Explanation: Engaging in ongoing education reflects lifelong learning and professional excellence. Compliance and obligation suggest external motivation, while time management organizes tasks. Continuous learning ensures competency and adaptability.

Q641. Answer: A

Explanation: Advocating for policy updates shows leadership by promoting evidence-based improvements. Delegation assigns duties, and compliance or control enforce existing rules. Leadership drives innovation, elevating patient care and professional standards.

Q642. Answer: D

Explanation: Transactional leaders motivate performance through rewards and recognition. Transformational leaders inspire vision, while autocratic and passive leaders limit engagement. Transactional methods reinforce accountability and measurable results.

Q643. Answer: A

Explanation: Research integrity demands unbiased data handling and ethical accuracy. Efficiency and adherence ensure process but not validity. Integrity ensures credibility, transparency, and professional responsibility in evidence generation.

Q644. Answer: A

Explanation: Holistic practice integrates physical, emotional, and social factors influencing health. Bias undermines fairness, administrative focus limits perspective, and legal compliance ensures regulation but not holistic care. Considering determinants promotes equity and wellness.

Q645. Answer: A

Explanation: Active listening is central to therapeutic communication, ensuring empathy and understanding. Detachment and task focus ignore emotional needs, while directive counseling limits expression. Listening fosters trust and patient-family support.

Q646. Answer: C

Explanation: Objectivity ensures evaluations are based on observable facts rather than opinions or emotions. Loyalty and avoidance distort fairness. Maintaining impartiality enhances credibility and developmental outcomes in peer review.

Q647. Answer: A

Explanation: Inclusivity values varied viewpoints, strengthening teamwork and innovation. Authority imposes direction, passive leadership neglects engagement, and competition divides teams. Inclusive collaboration improves morale and comprehensive care delivery.

Q648. Answer: A

Explanation: Surveillance responsibility involves recognizing and reporting potential outbreaks promptly. Delegation and compliance follow directives, not proactive identification. Reporting ensures timely intervention and patient safety.

Q649. Answer: C

Explanation: Highlighting positive ethics models professional behavior and motivates others. Promotion and favoritism distort fairness, and passive recognition lacks public encouragement. Role modeling sustains ethical culture and morale.

Q650. Answer: A

Explanation: Reflective practice involves self-assessment to enhance competence and professional growth. Task review focuses on completion, not insight. Supervision and administrative evaluation assess others, not self. Reflection fosters accountability and continual improvement.

Made in United States
Orlando, FL
04 November 2026

90201049R00087